PSYCHIATRIC DRUGS

A DESK REFERENCE

PSYCHIATRIC DRUGS

A DESK REFERENCE

Gilbert Honigfeld

Clinical Research Department
Sandoz Pharmaceuticals
Hanover, New Jersey

Alfreda Howard

Research Department—Hillside Division
Long Island Jewish—Hillside Medical Center
Glen Oaks, New York

 1973

ACADEMIC PRESS   New York   San Francisco   London
A Subsidiary of Harcourt Brace Jovanovich, Publishers

ACADEMIC PRESS, INC.
111 Fifth Avenue, New York, New York 10003

United Kingdom Edition published by
ACADEMIC PRESS, INC. (LONDON) LTD.
24/28 Oval Road, London NW1

LIBRARY OF CONGRESS CATALOG CARD NUMBER: 72-88360

PRINTED IN THE UNITED STATES OF AMERICA

CONTENTS

PREFACE

This book was written to meet the need for a multidisciplinary reference work on the clinical uses of psychiatric drugs. Psychologists, social workers, occupational therapists, psychiatric nurses, and other mental health professionals have had no desk reference to which they could turn for clear, nontechnical guidelines to current psychopharmacologic practice. Although several comprehensive medical texts on clinical psychopharmacology are available, these are not satisfactory for nonmedical clinicians. While they incorporate a significant amount of detailed and academic material, these medically oriented texts often lack the explicit clinical focus needed by the mental health professional.

In order to provide optimal patient care and guidance, it is now necessary for mental health workers of all disciplines to understand the basic indications and contraindications for psychiatric drug therapy. Recognizing when a patient needs psychiatric drug treatment and knowing how to evaluate such treatment are necessary skills for all mental health professionals. The nonmedical practitioner must understand that a vested interest

in a particular set of professional services should not blind him
to other, potentially helpful forms of treatment. It becomes particularly important to disseminate information about psychiatric
drugs, since they are so widely used and misused. Training in the
principles of psychiatric drug therapy is deficient. Few professional
schools offer courses in this area, and what little clinical psychopharmacology is acquired is usually picked up in a hit-or-miss
manner. This is understandable in that drugs can be prescribed
only by physicians. However, as nonmedical mental health professionals assume greater treatment responsibilities, their need for
knowledge about the potentials of all treatment modalities becomes increasingly apparent.

The material in this book is presented in a concise, nontheo-
retical manner. Although a relatively short volume, it contains a
great deal of information. The reader will find major sections
dedicated to each class of psychiatric drugs, as well as such topics
as side effects, current developments, and electroshock therapy.
Of special interest are Appendixes 1–7 which include trade and
generic drug name lists, and drug identification tables.

Drug product identification has been obtained from a variety
of sources and was accurate according to the authors' determination up to April 1972. Recommendations concerning dosage represent the authors' evaluation of current standards of good practice.
In some cases this may differ somewhat from the dosage ranges
recommended by the drug manufacturers. Academic Press as-
sumes no responsibility for these recommendations, which have
been determined solely by the authors.

ACKNOWLEDGMENTS

The manuscript for this book benefited considerably from the criticisms provided by a number of colleagues: George Bailis, M.D., Nathan S. Kline, M.D., Ann Mellers, Ph.D., Russell R. Monroe, M.D., Myron Pulier, M.D., Gary Rosenberg, M.S.W., and Paul Silverman, Ph.D.

Special thanks are due to Arthur Rifkin, M.D., who used an earlier draft of the book in teaching principles of psychopharmacology to nonmedical staff at Long Island Jewish–Hillside Medical Center. His thoughtful comments resulted in significant improvements in the text.

The authors' burden was considerably eased through the seemingly tireless efforts and endless good humor of two top-notch secretaries: Shirley De Bonis and Roslyn Siegel. Vivian Gualano and her secretarial staff at Rockland State Hospital deserve special thanks for their help. Thea Fenichel shared in the tedium of proofreading.

Finally, we acknowledge our special debt to Donald F. Klein, M.D. His research in psychopharmacology, particularly exploring the relationships between diagnosis and drug response has provided the principal theoretical orientation of this work. Because of the close professional relationships between the authors and Dr. Klein, his ideas have found their way onto many of the pages that follow. We hope our debt to him will be paid in part through extending the community of mental health professionals familiar with these ideas.

This work was made possible in part by support provided by Long Island Jewish-Hillside Medical Center (NIMH General Research Support Grant#FR5494), and Rockland (New York) State Hospital (NIMH Grant #14934).

CHAPTER 1

INTRODUCTION

Modern psychopharmacology, while less than 20 years old, has had a profound effect on the care and treatment of the mentally ill. Psychotic and affectively disturbed patients now have available to them a wide range of chemotherapeutic agents which, in many cases, hold the promise of significant relief from distress and decreased risk of relapse.

Information on developments of psychopharmacology has not been a significant part of the professional preparation of nonmedical mental health workers. This may reflect professional jealousy, or simply a feeling that psychopharmacology is of medical concern only and, therefore, is given a low priority in training. However, it is our view that such information should be a cornerstone of the professional preparation of every mental health worker for if the goal of clinical work is the patient's welfare, then the treatments offered should be the ones required. This is true even if those required treatments are not techniques for which the mental health worker is himself trained or legally licensed to administer. Using careful diagnostic study, the mental health professional should be concerned with each patient's total therapeutic needs and, when necessary, seek appropriate consultation. Frequently, this will mean

1

collaboration with a physician in order to review possible medication needs. Such patient-serving referrals can be made only if mental health professionals are aware of the indications for drug treatment.

This book is not an encyclopedic review of the psychopharmacology literature. Excellent scholarly reviews can be found elsewhere (Klein and Davis, 1969; Ban, 1969; Clark and del Giudice, 1970; Rech and Moore, 1971). Rather, we hope to provide a balanced overview of the current state of the clinical psychopharmacological arts from the point of view of the nonmedical mental health practitioner and student. Specifically, this book will be useful to psychologists, social workers, occupational therapists, psychiatric nurses, pastoral counsellors, and others in related professions.

The clinical indications, contraindications, and side effects of antidepressant, antipsychotic, antianxiety, and antimanic agents, as well as the sedative and activating drugs, and electroconvulsive therapy are reviewed. Included also is material on side effects, maintenance and preventive medication, drug treatment of drug abuse and alcoholism, new developments in drug treatment, and the management of drug emergencies. We hope that Chapter 14, "Evaluating Your Medical Colleagues," will be useful, keeping in mind that one day a psychiatrist may write a similar essay on "Evaluating Your Nonmedical Colleagues." A concluding chapter presents our views concerning the implications of this new field of psychopharmacology for mental health training in general.

Appendixes 1 and 2 enable the reader to translate between drug trade names and generic (chemical) names when reading the professional literature or when dealing with patients and their treatment histories.

Appendix 3 summarizes the physical appearance of psychoactive capsules and tablets organized according to trade name. This can be useful in corroborating patients' drug histories, particularly when the reliability of information may be in question. The necessary material is now available for reference when the worker asks a patient such a question as: "You mentioned that you thought you had been taking Elavil; do you remember what the pills looked like?"

Appendixes 4 and 5 will help establish drug identification through physical characteristics of the drugs alone, including form (tablet or capsule), color, shape, and special identifying marks. Information on tablets is in Appendix 4, and capsule information is in Appendix 5. These may be helpful when a patient cannot recall the name of a former medication, but does recall its appearance. Tables 4 and 5 may be especially valuable references during drug crises such as suicide attempts or accidental overdoses.

These reference tables refer principally to North American trade names and products; thus, their utility in other countries may be limited. These tables will be reviewed periodically to take account of new products, discontinuation of old products, and changes in the physical characteristics of the capsules and tablets.

Like much of medicine, psychopharmacology is largely an empirical science, with its most significant discoveries having been serendipitous. Many allied professionals have been unjustly critical of this. Certainly no one questions the use of quinine for malaria or penicillin for infections because these discoveries were accidental. The successes and failures in psychopharmacology have been more carefully detailed and researched than those in any other type of psychological or psychiatric treatment. Therefore, while psychopharmacology is still short on theory, it is long on supporting research, often of high quality. Ignore, if you will, the fact that the initial use of chlorpromazine was as a presurgical sedative; or that the antidepressant qualities of monoamine oxidase inhibitors were observed secondary to experimentation with tuberculosis suppressants; or that the "calming" effect of lithium on mice (leading to the suggestion that the drug be tried with manic patients) was nothing other than lithium-induced coma due to near-toxic doses. That significant therapeutic discoveries may be fortuitous should neither obscure nor diminish the quality of subsequent clinical investigations or the very profound effects that these drugs have had on the nature and quality of current psychiatric practice.

CHAPTER 2

ANTIDEPRESSANT DRUGS

The development of the antidepressant drugs, sometimes referred to as "psychic energizers" or "thymoleptics," represents one of the outstanding successes of modern psychopharmacology. The indications of drug treatment in serious affective disturbance are clear, and the expectation of a high incidence of favorable therapeutic response is justifiably great. Therefore, conscientious clinicians of all disciplines should be familiar with these facts so that appropriate consultations or referrals can be made. Numerous well-controlled studies attest to the efficacy of these drugs in combating depression and panic anxiety (e.g., Klerman and Paykel, 1970; Overall *et al.*, 1962).

Potential candidates for antidepressant drug treatment include patients with recurrent agitated or retarded depressions, as well as a group of phobic individuals who experience unexplained panic attacks. This emphasis on the role of chemotherapy does not mean that depressed and panic-anxious patients do not require psychological and environmental support. Usually, these patients suffer from associated feelings of inadequacy and demoralization and may require considerable psychotherapeutic support and counselling. On the other hand, in treating many depressed patients, one should think *first* of the possibility of an active antidepressant drug treatment program as one of the essential features of total treatment planning.

Depressions generally tend to lift spontaneously. Therefore, in the absence of well-controlled studies, it is easy for clinicians to take credit for a "cure," regardless of the type of treatment offered, as long as the patient improves. The self-limiting nature of most affective disturbances has tended to obscure the indications for somatic treatment, although many workers in this field feel that somatic treatment may accelerate the natural course of recovery in depression. The number of suicides prevented and amount of patient anguish alleviated by these treatment methods cannot be overestimated.

The two major categories of antidepressant drugs are: (*a*) the tricyclic group, of which imipramine (Tofranil) and amitriptyline (Elavil) are the most widely used, and (*b*), the monoamine oxidase (MAO) inhibitors, of which tranylcypromine (Parnate) and phenelzine (Nardil) are the best known. Principal members of these drug classes are presented in Table 2.1, along with typical therapeutic dose ranges. Less popular members of the antidepressant group are noted in Table 2.2.

The tricyclics, which are used more frequently in the United States, are discussed more fully below than are the MAO inhibitors. During the 1960s certain MAO inhibitors were implicated in several fatalities. For this reason, the entire class of MAO inhibitors fell into disuse. This was not the case in Europe where they are used at least as frequently as the tricyclics, with excellent results.

Indications

The classic indication for antidepressant medication is retarded depression; however, these drugs are also useful in the treatment of agitated depressions and phobic anxiety states, all of which are discussed below.

TABLE 2.1. ANTIDEPRESSANT DRUGS AND EFFECTIVE DOSAGE RANGES

Drug class	Generic name	Trade name	Effective adult daily dose ranges (mg)		
			High	Moderate	Low
Tricyclics	Amitriptyline	Elavil	225–300	150–225	50–150
	Desipramine	Norpramin Pertofrane	200–250	150–200	100–150
	Doxepin	Sinequan	225–300	150–225	50–150
	Imipramine	Tofranil	225–300	150–225	50–150
	Nortriptyline	Aventyl	100–150	75–100	50–75
	Protriptyline	Vivactil	45–60	30–45	15–30
MAO Inhibitors	Isocarboxazid	Marplan	40–60	20–40	10–20
	Pargyline	Eutonyl	75–100	50–75	25–50
	Phenelzine	Nardil	45–75	30–45	15–30
	Tranylcypromine	Parnate	30–40	20–30	10–20

6

TABLE 2.2. ADDITIONAL ANTIDEPRESSANTS

Drug class	Generic name	Trade name	Comment
Tricyclic	Opipramol	Ensidon	—
	Trimipramine	Surmontil	—
MAO Inhibitor	Etryptamine	Monase	Withdrawn from market because
	Iproniazid	Marsilid	of serious side effects
	Mebanazine	Actomol	—
	Nialamide	Niamid	Discontinued

RETARDED DEPRESSION

Central to all types of depression is a loss of ability to experience pleasure, associated with feelings of personal incompetence. Lack of interest, listlessness, somatic complaints, appetite, libido, and sleep disturbances, and suicidal ideation are frequent in all depressions. Outstanding in the retarded depressive is psychomotor slowing in which the patient appears unable to respond spontaneously at a normal speed, manifesting weak voice, labored speech, fixed facial expression, deliberate body movements, and slowed, dragging gait.

Childhood histories are usually unremarkable, with many patients having been good, well-behaved children, often well-liked by others. Early personality patterns vary widely among patients, and there seems to be no uniform type of childhood background associated with the development of subsequent affective disorder. Although it is possible that there may be a somewhat greater degree of infant separation anxiety in depressed patients than in other groups (Heinicke, 1970), this in itself does not appear to be diagnostic.

The onset of retarded depression may be insidious or abrupt, with many patients reporting it impossible to define any clear-cut transition in mood. However, an outstanding feature of all affective disorder is its periodicity. Most depressed patients tend to have cyclic histories with more than one similar episode. Although some may have predictable cycles, for many it is usually impossible to predict the time at which an affective disturbance will return. In general, symptoms of depressions tend to be self-limiting; when untreated, however, the episode may take months or several years to resolve itself.

Prompt intervention with antidepressants at adequate dosages seems to accelerate the natural recovery process. An important point affecting case management is that antidepressant drugs (tricyclics, in particular) require at least two weeks before therapeutic effects emerge. Therefore, patients may need extensive support to help them through this difficult waiting period. Dosage should be increased regularly. Using imipramine (Tofranil) as the standard example, an initial, daily adult oral dosage of 75 mg, increased slowly to as high as 225–300 mg daily within 2–3 weeks should be instituted. The treatment plan should include a 1-month trial period at full-dosage level, during which time signs of drug response should be seen. If, at the end of this period no therapeutic response is found despite the administration of maximum dosage for three weeks, the patient should be switched to another class of antidepressant drugs (that is, the MAO inhibitors), or his diagnosis be reconsidered. In no case should a patient be allowed to drift on an ineffective drug for more than a month.

On the other hand, case management during the initial 2–3 weeks of antidepressant treatment may be particularly difficult since the patient and his family will require considerable support in order to continue with the prescribed medication in the absence of quick, favorable response. A positive attitude toward drug treatment can be fostered by the mental health worker since there is, in fact, a very high likelihood of ultimate therapeutic benefit. It is essential, however, that the patient and family members understand at the outset that antidepressant medication will not produce an overnight cure. Patients and families may need to be instructed that early signs of progress can include such things as appetite increase and improved sleep patterns prior to the patient's report of improved mood.

AGITATED DEPRESSION

Antidepressant drugs are also indicated in the treatment of agitated depression. As with retarded depression, patients with agitated depressions also show a loss of ability to experience pleasure, as well as associated feelings of incompetence. However, in opposition to the motor inhibition of the retarded depressive, the agitated patient seems to share with the manic an excess of motor activity, including such characteristically unproductive behaviors as handwringing, incessant pacing, and monotonous complaining.

Other diagnostic clues to agitated depression include a very demanding aspect in the patient–therapist relationship, unrestrained expressions of emotion, restless, accelerated behavior, and obsessive, unpleasant ruminations. The premorbid histories of such patients frequently involve obsessional life-styles with stereotyped, repetitive, unadventuresome patterns. In this regard, they resemble other obsessional individuals who never develop agitated depressive disorders. Agitated depressions often present a cyclic pattern with unpredictable, repeated episodes occurring throughout adult life, with good psychosocial functioning between episodes. It is also common for agitated depressions to occur for the first time during late middle age (the involutional period), often with abrupt onset.

In attempting to make the differential diagnosis, one should remember that a relatively long-lasting depression can be precipitated by life events. Therefore, despite an understandable psychological "trigger" for the depression, drug therapy may still be a highly effective treatment. Besides bereavement, possible precipitants of retarded or agitated depressions include viral and bacterial infections, prolonged fatigue, debilitation and weight loss, surgery, endocrine disorders, disappointment or feelings of psychological loss. The use of certain drugs for either psychiatric or medical purposes [e.g., the use of steroids, or reserpine (Serpasil) for the treatment of high blood pressure] can produce abnormal psychological states, including precipitating a depression. Therefore, it is very important to take careful drug histories as part of the total patient-evaluation process.

As will be discussed in the next chapter, some antipsychotic agents are also useful in treating agitated depressions, with equally good expectations of therapeutic results. Because these drugs have a more immediate effect on the motor acceleration features of the disorder, many psychiatrists will prefer this form of treatment. This is an entirely reasonable procedure, particularly during the acute stage when features of agitation may be very pronounced.

Because agitated depressions are common in involutional and geriatric patients, and because antidepressant drugs may have hypotensive side effects (reduced blood pressure), the question of each patient's cardiovascular status must be evaluated prior to the prescription of antidepressant medication. Furthermore, patients who are grossly underweight, physically debilitated, or suffering serious medical illness, may require lower dosage levels to reduce the risks of toxicity. On the other hand, few patients are found medically unsuitable for psychotropic medication when this is indicated by their psychiatric conditions.

Comprehensive management of the drug-treated, depressed patient usually involves psychotherapy and counseling. However, it should be kept in mind that during the acute phase of the patient's illness, exploratory psychotherapy tends to be ineffective because of the patient's low ego strength and general feelings of incompetence. It is frequently necessary to take a directive hand in managing the patient's life, to structure his activities as much as possible in order to prevent further withdrawal, brooding or depressive or suicidal preoccupations. It is important to attempt to get such a patient involved in any kind of activity which may serve to distract him from his preoccupations. Easily accomplished, goal-directed tasks are ideal and can include such simple routines as washing dishes and making beds: depressed patients should not be allowed simply to vegetate. Later, as the patient begins to move through the resolving phase of the illness into the maintenance stage, more explorative psychotherapy may be considered.

PANIC ANXIETY

The antidepressants (particularly the tricyclics, e.g., imipramine) are also indicated in the treatment of panic anxiety where the individual suffers from recurrent, unexplained, panic attacks, with feelings of impending doom and associated physical symptoms such as heart palpitations and breathing difficulties. These dramatic, incapacitating symptoms usually occur spontaneously, with no apparent external stimulus, although such factors as moving to a new home may be expected to trigger panic attacks in the susceptible, separation-sensitive individual. Often the onset of panic anxiety is at a time of disturbed endocrine function such as after childbirth, after a hysterectomy, or at menopause. The attacks are frequently associated with specific fear-producing situations—being in crowded stores or meeting strangers. This results in a prominent phobic overlay in such a patient's psychopathology.

An underlying fear seems to be the feeling that there may be no help at hand when an unexpected panic attack occurs. Such patients, therefore, may be unable to leave their home unless accompanied by a family member or friend; crossing a street or using public transportation may be impossible. This disorder frequently becomes the central focus of the patient's life, rendering him completely incapable of working productively except within the confines of his own home (Klein and Davis, 1969).

Because of the extreme discomfort characteristic of this disorder, attempts at self-medication are quite common; many patients turn to barbiturates or alcohol as a means of obtaining temporary relief. These agents are moderately effective, particularly when used to the point of "feeling no pain." Therefore, problems of drug and alcohol abuse are common sequelae to this disorder. In evaluating the case history of an alcoholic or drug abuser, it is important to determine whether there might not be a primary panic-anxiety disorder which is being hidden by the more prominent symptoms of drug or alcohol abuse.

With imipramine (Tofranil) treatment, almost all such patients lose their panic attacks completely or experience a significant reduction in the intensity and frequency of attacks. In terms of drug management, patients in this diagnostic group are treated similarly to depressed patients, but with favorable responses coming at lower dosage levels. Imipramine should be started at 25 mg daily, increasing 25 mg daily until 150 mg daily is reached. Rarely is a higher dosage necessary.

However, antidepressants alone, which may help reduce or eliminate the panic experiences per se, generally do not in themselves represent a total treatment program. These patients tend to develop an overlay of anticipatory anxiety; that is, even when the panic attacks subside, the patient may remain morbidly preoccupied with the possibility that should he venture from home he might be helpless were he to have a panic attack. This secondary, anticipatory anxiety can be treated with counseling, psychotherapy, behavior therapy, or the use of antianxiety drugs (see Chapter 4). Combined therapeutic efforts (e.g., drugs and psychotherapy) aimed at ridding a patient of his overlay of anticipatory anxiety are possible, and may prove ultimately to be more demanding of therapeutic skills than the initial problem of reducing or eliminating the actual panic attacks.

Family counseling is usually an essential part of the total treatment program, to insure that family members offer the patient an appropriate blend of psychological support without infantilization.

Contraindications

Antidepressants are generally not indicated in treating acute schizophrenia, where their use is often associated with exacerbation of symptoms. Occasionally, use of antidepressants in modest dosages during the residual phase of schizophrenic disorders is useful when apathy is present, secondary to phenothiazine use. This treatment must be carefully monitored for signs of re-emergent symptomatology which could result from overuse of antidepressants in schizophrenic patients.

Except for the special indication of monoamine oxidase (MAO) inhibitors for certain patients with hysterical character disorders (see Chapter 11), antidepressant drugs are of little value in treating neurotic and character disorder patients.

Side Effects

Because the use of antidepressants is sometimes associated with the appearance of side effects, unskilled practitioners may err by prescribing drugs at low dosage levels. In light of the rather serious nature of most affective disorders, this could be a significant therapeutic error: most depressed patients require treatment at the upper end of the indicated therapeutic ranges before benefits are seen; this, in turn, maximizes the likelihood of unwanted side effects.

In prescribing psychotropic drugs, the skillful psychiatrist will usually try to keep side reactions to a minimum by using gradual build-up periods. This allows the patient to adapt physiologically to the new chemical. At the same time, however, he will continue to build to fairly high dosage levels in order to maximize therapeutic benefits. Within reasonable limits, he may justifiably continue to do this in the face of tolerable side effects.

Of course, there are many exceptions to this rule. Because of possible hypotensive (lowered blood pressure) side effects of antidepressant medication, patients with cardiovascular problems are usually treated at lower dosage ceilings than other patients. Elderly, debilitated patients are also often drug-sensitive and require reduced dosages.

With the MAO inhibitors, cerebrovascular effects may be particularly troublesome. Patients should be carefully instructed to avoid foods such as aged cheeses and wines which may be high in tyramine (a fermentation by-product). In combination with MAO inhibitor drugs, these foods may produce potentially lethal hypertensive crises. Therefore, everyone having clinical responsibilities for patients on MAO inhibitors should be alert to signs of increased blood pressure such as:

1. Severe, atypical headaches (which may radiate from the back of the head forward)
2. Heart palpitations
3. Neck stiffness
4. Sweating
5. Cold, clammy skin
6. Dilated pupils
7. Chest pain
8. Rapid heart rate
9. Slow heart rate

Appendix 6 is a rather complete reference list of foods high in tyramine which should be avoided by patients on MAO inhibitors.

The MAO inhibitors are also incompatible with certain other drugs, especially stimulants, cold tablets, and reducing pills. Such medicines can represent a serious hazard to the patient on MAO inhibitors, and their use should be at the discretion of the physician only. Another hazard is the novocaine used by dentists which usually contains epinephrine (adrenalin). The dentist should be told that a patient is taking MAO inhibitors so he can use pure novocaine, novocaine plus norepinephrine, or "cardiac" novocaine.

A more complete catalog of potential antidepressant drug side effects is given in Chapter 8. It should be apparent from our discussion of side effects that psychotropic drugs are not innocuous preparations, but have certain hazards associated with their use. Furthermore, psychotropic drug prescriptions cannot be based exclusively on the patient's psychiatric status—his total medical condition must be considered.

CHAPTER 3

ANTIPSYCHOTIC AGENTS

The antipsychotic agents, frequently referred to as major tranquilizers, psycholeptics, or neuroleptics, are highly effective in the treatment of a number of specific psychological disturbances. At the same time, these drugs are widely misused by both psychiatrists and general medical practitioners unfamiliar with the appropriate indications for their use. Their indiscriminate overuse has been fostered by the drug manufacturers, in part, by their unfortunate early categorization of these drugs as "tranquilizers," implying that their principal application is in the treatment of anxiety states. Under careful investigation, this has been found to be untrue (Brill *et al.*, 1964; Smith and Chassan, 1964; Vilkin, 1964).

The antipsychotic agents include four major classes of drugs: phenothiazines, butyrophenones, thioxanthenes, and reserpines. The reserpines, because they are less effective and more toxic, are no longer used in psychiatric treatment. All major phenothiazines, butyrophenones, and thioxanthenes commercially available in the United States are listed in Table 3.1, with typical, effective adult dosage ranges. It will be seen in Table 3.1 that there are wide dif-

TABLE 3.1. MAJOR ANTIPSYCHOTIC AGENTS AND EFFECTIVE DOSAGE RANGES

Drug class and type	Generic name	Trade name(s)	Effective adult daily dose ranges (mg)		
			High	Moderate	Low
Soporific phenothiazines	Chlorpromazine	Thorazine Largactil	800–2000	400–800	50–400
	Promazine	Sparine	600–1200	200–600	40–200
	Thioridazine	Mellaril	600–1000	400–600	75–400
	Triflupromazine	Vesprin	120–200	100–150	50–100
Nonsoporific phenothiazines	Acetophenazine	Tindal	60–80	40–60	20–40
	Fluphenazine	Permitil Prolixin	10–20	5–10	1–5
	Perphenazine	Trilafon	40–64	24–40	8–24
	Prochlorperazine	Compazine	90–150	60–90	15–60
	Trifluoperazine	Stelazine	20–40	10–20	2–10
Butyrophenones	Haloperidol	Haldol, Serenace	10–15	6–10	2–6
Thioxanthenes	Thiothixene	Navane	48–60	24–48	6–24
	Chlorprothixene	Solatron, Taractan	800–2000	400–800	75–400

16

ferences in effective dose ranges within this drug class. These differences are the result of molecular variations in the compounds, but the dose ranges given represent approximately equivalent levels in terms of expected clinical responses. The dose ranges noted as *high* sometimes exceed manufacturer's recommendations but are consistent with current models of good practice. It is most common

TABLE 3.2. ADDITIONAL ANTIPSYCHOTIC AGENTS

Generic name	Trade name(s)	Drug class	Manufacturer
Acepromazine	Notensil, Plegicil	Phenothiazine	Clin-Byla
Butaperazine	Repoise	Phenothiazine	Robins
Carphenazine	Proketazine	Phenothiazine	Wyeth
Clopenthixol	Sordinol	Phenothiazine	Ayerst
Dehydrobenzperidol	Innovar	Butyrophenone	McNeil
Dixyrazine	Esucos	Phenothiazine	Union Chimiques Belge
Mepazine	Pacatal	Phenothiazine	Warner
Mesoridazine	Serentil	Phenothiazine	Sandoz
Methophenazine	Frenelon	Phenothiazine	Medimpex
Methotrimeprazine	Levoprome Veractil Nirvan	Phenothiazine	Lederle May & Baker United Drug
Methoxypromazine	Tentone	Phenothiazine	Lederle
Pipamazine	Mornidine	Phenothiazine	Searle
Piperacetazine	Quide	Phenothiazine	Pitman-Moore
Promethazine	Phenergan	Phenothiazine	Wyeth
Propericiazine	Neuleptil	Phenothiazine	Rhone-Poulenc
Propiomazine	Largon	Phenothiazine	Wyeth
Thiazinamium	Multergan	Phenothiazine	Rhone-Poulenc
Thiethylperazine	Torecan	Phenothiazine	Sandoz
Thiopropazate	Dartal	Phenothiazine	Searle
Thioproperazine	Majeptil	Phenothiazine	Rhone-Poulenc
Xanthiol	Daxid	Thioxanthene	Pfizer

for patients to be treated with *high* doses in in-patient settings, where the increased chance of side effects can be adequately monitored. Less widely used members of these drug classes are indicated in Table 3.2.

Of these drug classes, the most important are the phenothiazines, being the most widely used clinically and the best-studied experimentally. Table 3.1 shows the major phenothiazines classified as *soporific* (sedating) and *nonsoporific*. The reader should be aware, however, that there are wide differences among individuals in their susceptibility to the possibly sedating effects of psychotropic drugs.

The major indication for these compounds is in treating the various forms of schizophrenia; they are also useful in the treatment of agitated depressive states and emotionally unstable personalities (Klein and Davis, 1969).

Introduced into American psychiatric practice in the mid-1950s, the use of these drugs was associated almost immediately with a decrease in hospital populations and the opening of many closed custodial wards. This coincided closely with the efforts of humanistically oriented social scientists to open the mental hospital more fully to the community and convert institutional policies from custodial care to active therapeutic programs. Under both these influences, dramatic gains were made in the treatment of schizophrenia during the 1960s. It is now possible to treat many patients in the community, with the expectation that some can quickly be returned to their premorbid status. These developments have made the implementation of the community mental health center concept much more feasible.

Schizophrenia

Few clinical areas are as confused or controversial as the concept of "schizophrenia." Some feel that this is a catch-all category, so broad and vaguely defined that any eccentric individual is labeled "schizophrenic." Others reject this label, substituting instead a behavioral analysis unique to each individual. Still others feel that while individual manifestations of associative disturbance or delusional thinking may vary widely from patient to patient, nonetheless, the presence of certain core abnormalities point to a valid, clinical category. Five diagnostic traits are common to schizophrenia in all its forms (although not all, of course, may be present in any single patient):

1. Hallucinations
2. Delusions
3. Thought disorder
4. Emotional disorder
5. Motor disturbance

Hallucinations are perceptual experiences in the absence of corresponding sensory stimuli. While hallucinations may occur in any sense modality, it is the auditory form which is most characteristic of schizophrenia. Visual, olfactory, gustatory, and tactile hallucinations are much more suggestive of organic, or hysterical disorders.

Delusions are unjustified beliefs which may develop as part of the schizophrenic's attempt to explain his perceptual distortions and misevaluations. The development of such erroneous beliefs is usually accompanied by inner feelings of keen insight and revelation and, therefore, have the force of reality. The schizophrenic usually holds his delusions firmly and cannot be "talked out of" his delusion. Much delusional thinking is of a highly personalized nature, where apparently innocuous events are perceived as having special relevance for the patient. Such self-aggrandizing thinking is common in schizophrenia. Paranoid delusions refer to self-referential beliefs in the persecutory intent of other individuals toward the patient.

Thought disorder refers to the frequently observed peculiarities in schizophrenics' communicative abilities and inferential reasoning. While many varieties of thinking disturbance are possible, features seen frequently in schizophrenia include blocking and disappearance of thoughts, use of neologisms, and inability to focus attention.

However, the presence of these symptoms does not necessarily ensure a diagnosis of schizophrenia.

Emotional disorders, including emotional blunting and flatness of affect, are quite characteristic of the schizophrenic disorder. Inappropriate affect, where there is clear incongruity of thought and affect, is also diagnostic of schizophrenia. A wide range of emotional states found in schizophrenics includes intense anger, fear, and states of elation and depression, but these are not specific to this diagnostic group.

Motor disturbances in schizophrenia include the assumption of awkward and bizarre postures, as well as waxy flexibility, and occasionally stuporous states. Inappropriate smiling, grimacing, mutism, and repeated behavioral rituals are also reported in schizophrenia, as are states of wild excitement. For some reason, such motor signs were more prevalent in the 19th century than they are at present. These signs cannot be considered entirely diagnostic in themselves; patients with certain affective, hysterical, and organic disorders may also have similar motor peculiarities.

Psychosis has been defined as "a persistent misevaluation of perception, which has the force of reality, and which is not attributable to sensory defect or afferent abnormality" (Klein and Davis, 1969, p.33). Therefore, a diagnostic evaluation for schizophrenia must rule out other possible causes of psychosis such as infection, toxic states, physical trauma, seizure disorder, cerebral tumor, cerebrovascular disease, senile degeneration, or metabolic disturbances. Certain temporary factors which may produce psychotic manifestations include loss of sleep, battle stress, drug and alcohol abuse, and states of sensory deprivation. In addition, some manic-depressive and hysterical patients may be hard to distinguish from schizophrenics.

A Kraepelinian diagnostic model of schizophrenia is followed here, where the diagnosis is based not only on presenting symptomatology, but on an evaluation of the patient's past history and course of illness as well. The goal of such evaluation is to arrive at a diagnostic classification with predictive utility for either: (*a*) predicting the course of the illness if untreated, or (*b*) predicting possible outcome given available treatment methods.

This approach makes diagnosis much more than an academic exercise, since with proper diagnosis, treatment planning can be made more efficient and reliable. Anticipating a more complete consideration later in this chapter, three schizophrenic subtypes whose differential responses to medication can generally be predicted accurately are (*a*) "process" schizophrenia—patients with a significant history of childhood asociality, (*b*) paranoid schizophrenia—where symptoms generally begin to appear in adolescence, and (*c*) "reactive" or schizo-affective schizophrenia (Klein and Davis, 1969).

This brief overview of schizophrenic symptomatology is presented to provide some uniformity in discussing the major schizophrenic subtypes with established relationships to drug effects and overall prognosis.

"PROCESS" SCHIZOPHRENIA

In childhood, these patients were usually markedly deviant, aloof, asocial, and eccentric. Scapegoating by peers is a frequent feature, along with scholastic difficulty. During symptom episodes, these patients typically show thought disturbance with vague, disconnected speech and over-concrete or over-abstract thinking. Frequently they seek to deny or minimize their illness. Paranoid features may be present, but the delusional thought is often poorly formed and bizarre.

Among schizophrenics, the "process" patients are the most refractory to all types of treatment and have the poorest overall prognosis. According to the official APA diagnostic system (see Tables 13.1–13.5) such patients would usually be considered to have simple, hebephrenic, or catatonic schizophrenia.

PARANOID SCHIZOPHRENIA

These patients too have a poor long-term prognosis, although they may benefit somewhat from medication and counseling. During the acute phase of the illness they may exhibit many characteristics in common with the "process" group, with prominent suspiciousness and defensiveness. However, their delusions seem generally to be better-formed than those of schizophrenics with histories of childhood asociality. Auditory hallucinations and ideas of reference are common, and frequently relate to the belief that others are making derogatory or sexual comments about them. Furthermore, delusional ideas may concern the possibility of bodily change, particularly sexual inversion. Feelings of depression may be marked and suicidal preoccupations are reported, sometimes in response to hallucinated threats or commands. Outbursts of anger are common, usually in response to delusional distortions of reality.

The typical paranoid patient shows considerably less history of childhood deviance than does the "process" schizophrenic, although unfriendliness and social withdrawal are not uncommon. The illness tends to have its onset in adolescence, with a progressive deteriorative course. Initial psychotic episodes often occur in the 20s, and patients are usually diagnosed as having acute, paranoid, or catatonic schizophrenia, using the APA nomenclature (see Tables 13.1–13.5).

REACTIVE SCHIZOPHRENIA

This subgroup benefits most from psychotropic agents and has the most favorable long-term outcome. These patients closely resemble the manic-depressive patient. When excited, they show flight of ideas, hyperactivity, and possibly anger. In the retarded phase, such patients have psychomotor inhibition and appear depressed and unspontaneous. The diagnostic criteria which differentiate this group from manic-depressive patients relate to the presence of clear-cut delusions and hallucinations, with massive referential thinking and peculiar inferential processes.

Onset of illness is usually abrupt and occurs in young adulthood; childhood histories are usually unremarkable. Initial symptomatology may closely resemble the manic-depressive in that affective symptomatology is most prominent. When this is followed by severe cognitive and perceptual impairment, the differential diagnosis with manic-depressive psychosis is fairly straightforward. Under the APA nomenclature, such patients would generally be diagnosed schizo-affective.

Effectiveness of Antipsychotic Agents

Numerous controlled studies of the late 1950s and early 1960s attest to the utility of the antipsychotic agents in the treatment of schizophrenia. An able, comprehensive review of the extensive literature in this field can be found in Klein and Davis (1969).

A series of multihospital studies sponsored by the Veterans Administration probably served as models for the later controlled studies in psychopharmacology sponsored by the National Institute of Mental Health (Clark and del Giudice, 1970, Chap. 34) and other investigators. This series of investigations demonstrated conclusively the general effectiveness of the major antipsychotic agents in reducing symptomatology in schizophrenic patients (Casey *et al.*, 1960a; Casey *et al.*, 1961). A comparative study of various members of the same drug class also served to isolate the somewhat less effective members of the phenothiazine group (Casey *et al.*, 1960b). Having identified some of the weaker drugs in this class, attention turned to possible unique attributes of individual drugs (Caffey *et al.*, 1970).

Later, more refined studies designed to test the issue of selectivity of drug action for certain patient groups have been somewhat less successful. There is as yet little, well-controlled evidence bearing on the indications for one phenothiazine over another in the treatment of schizophrenic subgroups (Goldberg *et al.*, 1967; Klett and Moseley, 1965).

In terms of the general effects of phenothiazines on schizophrenic symptomatology, Table 3.3 provides a summary drawn from a number of reports, tabulating symptoms seen in schizophrenia and degree of expected positive effect.

Studies of Combined Drug and Social and Psychological Therapies

Although there have been only several comparative investigations in which drugs and psychotherapy were simultaneously

TABLE 3.3. SOME EFFECTS OF PHENOTHIAZINES
IN SCHIZOPHRENIC PATIENTS[a]

Schizophrenic symptom	Positive effect
Thinking disorder	Definite
Withdrawal	Definite
Autistic behavior	Definite
Hyperactivity	Definite
Uncooperativeness	Definite
Combativeness	Definite
Hallucinations	Probable
Paranoid ideation	Probable
Hostility	Probable
Mannerisms	Probable
Blunted affect	Possible
Depression	Possible
Disorientation	Minimal
Somatization	Minimal
Insight	Minimal

[a] After Klerman (1970) and Klein and Davis (1969).

studied, the evidence thus far fails to demonstrate that social or psychological therapies alone are of significant value for the schizophrenic patient. Drug effects consistently emerge as significant, with occasional supporting evidence that optimal treatment strategy incorporates drug treatment in a setting of active social or psychological intervention (Gorham and Pokorny, 1964; Greenblatt *et al.*, 1965; Grinspoon *et al.*, 1968; Honigfeld *et al.*, 1965; May, 1968).

General Treatment Considerations

Antipsychotic drug therapy of a schizophrenic patient should vary, depending upon the stage of the patient's illness, whether incipient, acute, resolving, or residual (Klein and Davis, 1969).

INCIPIENT SCHIZOPHRENIA

This is a difficult diagnostic discrimination to make since manifest symptoms of psychosis may not be present. Characteristic of this stage of the illness is affective lability, insomnia, bad dreams, agitation, perplexity, confusion, and feelings of depersonalization. Other symptoms may include alterations in social participation with gradual progressive isolation, suspiciousness, and social withdrawal. Frequently there is no clear line between these prodromal (early) states and the ultimate psychosis.

Because of the recent increase in toxic reactions related to drug abuse, it has become still more difficult to make the diagnosis of incipient schizophrenia. Marijuana, the amphetamines, and hallucinogens can all produce affective lability. Therefore, it is essential to detail the patient's history of drug use as completely and reliably as possible.

Current concepts of good practice include the prescription of antipsychotic agents to patients suspected of being in the incipient stage of a schizophrenic illness (APA diagnosis 295.5, latent schizo-phrenia). Because it is always in the patient's interest to try to pre-vent a full-blown psychotic episode, active chemotherapeutic intervention is clearly indicated.

Enlisting the family's cooperation in drug treatment is essential, since the patient himself often cannot be depended upon to follow the prescribed drug schedule. There is often a tendency on the part of both patient and family to minimize or deny difficulties as a means of demonstrating the patient's good health. The family must recognize, however, the importance of medication and not reject the use of prescribed drugs. Similarly, the mental health worker should not deny the seriousness of the patient's condition.

Phenothiazines, butyrophenones, or thioxanthenes in adequate dosages are indicated for such patients. Among the phenothiazines, mepazine (Pacatal), promazine (Sparine) and thiopropazate (Dartal) seem generally less effective than other members of this group. If insomnia is a problem, a soporific (sedative) phenothiazine may be prescribed, with the total daily drug dosage taken about an hour before retiring. The sedation threshold varies widely from patient to patient and consequently the soporific effects are hard to predict.

Typical dosage schedules begin at 100–200 mg, with daily incre-ments of 100 mg until the therapeutic range is reached. Therapeutic doses may be 600–1000 mg daily, possibly up to 2000 mg or more of chlorpromazine (Thorazine), in in-patient settings. Failure to treat patients at adequate dosage levels is a common therapeutic error. Chlorpromazine (Thorazine), the most well-known and widely used soporific phenothiazine, serves as the example; other antipsychotic agents may be used with equal success. While certain patients may develop idiosyncratic side effects to one or another antipsychotic drug, the physician would be wise to try a drug from another anti-psychotic class, rather than discontinue medication.

When the drugs are used at appropriate dosage levels, therapeutic response is expected within 4–6 weeks. If significant improvement has not occurred within this time period, diagnostic reevaluation should be considered. It should also be determined whether or not the patient has actually been taking the full dosage of medication.

Assuming the patient has made an adequate response, the question of long-term treatment planning naturally arises. Schizophrenia tends to be a chronic, recurrent illness, and there is evidence, based on the performance of chronic schizophrenic patients with long drug treatment histories, that withdrawal of antipsychotic medication is associated with greatly increased relapse rates (see Chapter 9). In the absence of data to the contrary, a conservative treatment approach includes long-term maintenance drug therapy for most patients with a history of schizophrenia. Many psychiatrists like to use a high potency, nonsoporific phenothiazine such as fluphenazine (Prolixin, Permitil), given in dosages of 2–10 mg daily, as the long-term maintenance medication for such patients. This dosage is within the therapeutic range but is usually low enough to prevent the appearance of significant side effects.

Despite diverse opinions about the etiology of schizophrenia, psychotherapeutic or counseling contacts can prove beneficial in helping such patients learn to deal with their adaptive difficulties. However, the psychotherapist should avoid grandiosity in his therapeutic planning for the patient, since there is no convincing evidence that psychotherapy alone has a prophylactic effect in recurrent psychosis. Clinically, one finds that many patients apparently recovered from earlier schizophrenic episodes may develop acute psychoses despite good family and social support. Others, on the contrary, may return to an unfavorable environment and remain relatively symptom-free.

Nevertheless, continued counseling contacts are desirable, both for helping the patient develop ego strength, as well as to monitor possible changes in clinical status so that, if necessary, active drug treatment can be reinstituted. Of particular significance in monitoring such patients is the appearance of atypical mood swings or increased social withdrawal. The appearance of such symptoms should be a signal for possible review of chemotherapy.

ACUTE SCHIZOPHRENIA

An initial decision that must be made when dealing with an *acute* schizophrenic psychosis is whether or not the patient is to be hospitalized. Despite the inadequacies of many psychiatric hospitals, as well as the social stigma associated with hospitalization and potential disruption of the patient's social milieu, it will frequently be impossible for the acute schizophrenic patient to be maintained outside a hospital setting. Furthermore, case management varies according to diagnostic subclassification, whether (a) "process," (b) paranoid, or (c) schizo-affective.

"Process" Schizophrenia. Despite their generally poor prognosis, of all acute schizophrenics, the childhood asocial, "process" patients are the easiest to maintain in the community. Their customary role in the family is parasitic, and since lessened social demands are usually made on these patients, it may be possible to maintain them out of the hospital during the acute stage. If their behavior becomes very bizarre, causing difficulties for family members, hospitalization may be unavoidable (Eveloff, 1970). A typical phenothiazine treatment regimen would include increasing daily doses of chlorpromazine (Thorazine), in 100 mg increments to the range of 600–1000 mg per day and perhaps higher. If sedation is not desired, a nonsoporific phenothiazine may be preferable. As treatment continues, patients may become less fearful, but may appear indifferent and apathetic. Delusional material may be less manifest and somatic complaints may increase. Despite the use of antiparkinson agents, these patients sometimes appear "zombie-like."

Paranoid Schizophrenia. Because the untreated paranoid patient is easily provoked to anger and is fearful, suspicious, and defensive, such patients are almost always hospitalized during the acute phase. Psychotic symptomatology is blatant, with ideas of reference, auditory hallucinations, delusional ideas, and frequently depression and suicidal preoccupation.

In-patient treatment regimens will frequently build up to the level of 2000 mg or more of chlorpromazine (Thorazine) daily, or its equivalent, with the expectation of only slight to moderate improvement. High dosage phenothiazine therapy should continue for 6–8 weeks, with adjunctive electro-convulsive therapy (ECT) as a possible therapeutic supplement.

Combination drug therapy may be indicated. If anticipatory anxiety is a subsidiary problem, an antianxiety agent such as chlordiazepoxide (Librium), 400–1000 mg daily, may help facilitate desirable social interaction (see Chapter 4).

Schizo-Affective Schizophrenia. Although a few such acutely ill patients are able to remain in the community, in general these patients are delusional and belligerent, and usually require close supervision. The excited schizo-affective patient requires very large doses of antipsychotic agents. Because of its fast action, the best practice seems to be initiating treatment with intramuscular chlorpromazine (Thorazine), perhaps 100 mg intramuscularly, three times daily. This can continue for two to three days, while liquid or oral phenothiazines are built up to 1500–2000 mg of chlorpromazine daily. At this time the intramuscular medication is discontinued. For excited patients, soporific phenothiazines such as chlorpromazine (Thorazine) or thioridazine (Mellaril) seem particularly useful. Due to the special dangers of side effects with thioridazine in daily dosages greater than 1000 mg (see Chapter 8), chlorpromazine is probably the drug of choice.

Because he causes little trouble, the schizo-affective patient with psychomotor retardation can occasionally be maintained in the community. These patients are frequently depressed and unspontaneous. The response of the retarded schizo-affective patient is more gradual than the excited patient, with a slow restoration of normal psychomotor rate and decreased suspiciousness and perplexity. Electro-convulsive therapy (ECT) can be considered with these patients if high dose phenothiazines have not been effective within 6–8 weeks (see Chapter 7).

RESOLVING PHASE

During the resolving phase of a schizophrenic illness, the patient may be greatly troubled by the realization that he has been so sick. He may feel overwhelmed by his social, familial, and economic situation; skilled counseling is thus necessary during this period. To encourage the development of adaptive strategies and a feeling of social effectiveness, familial support is especially crucial since the initial enthusiasm the family associates with the patient's symptomatic improvement may give way to an awareness of the patient's current limitations. The family members consequently may feel that they are being exploited and in some way reject the patient. Therefore, family therapy seems especially indicated at this time.

From a chemotherapeutic point of view, the most important issue would appear to be the determination of an adequate maintenance dose. Phenothiazine dosages equivalent to 300–600 mg chlorpromazine (Thorazine) daily are typical for this period. The psychiatrist may also wish at this stage to switch the patient to a nonsoporific phenothiazine. During the course of antipsychotic agent maintenance treatment, it is possible for a patient to become apathetic. A prompt response to a tricyclic antidepressant is not uncommon, in doses equal to 75–150 mg of imipramine (Tofranil) daily, concurrent with the phenothiazine. However, this can be a hazardous procedure since antidepressants may precipitate acute psychotic symptomatology in remitted schizophrenics. Concurrent antidepressant treatment should be carefully monitored for evidence of exacerbation of psychosis; this should be a relatively short-term intervention.

RESIDUAL SCHIZOPHRENIA

The residual characteristics of schizophrenia vary considerably among the three major groups. Following remission, "process" schizophrenics are still typically inept, inappropriate, bizarre, and dependent, with frequent evidences of thinking disturbance. They tend to be most comfortable with repetitive, simple routines but even with these may fatigue easily. Usually such patients occupy symbiotic social roles, whether in the hospital or at home, and long-term intensive psychotherapy is not usually expected to produce significant changes. Maintenance antipsychotic medication should probably be continued in light of its possible prophylactic effects, although it may require extensive encouragement on the part of both medical and nonmedical personnel to keep the patient on his prescribed drug regimen. In such cases, psychotherapy may be necessary to make the patient amenable to chemotherapy. Antidepressants should *not* be used in process schizophrenia (except for time-limited periods at low to moderate dosages), because these agents may possibly exacerbate further psychotic episodes. Schizophrenics who report visual hallucinations should be questioned concerning possible use of antidepressants. Day hospital placement provides a reasonable alternative to either full-time custodial care or full-time family responsibility for these patients. Activity and work programs sponsored by the day hospital can likely be oriented toward the patient's optimal emotional and cognitive level, with the advantage of continuous professional supervision and monitoring. The overall prognosis for "process" schizophrenia is poor, and with repeated psychotic episodes becomes poorer. This group of patients probably provides the bulk of permanently hospitalized, chronic schizophrenic patients.

At the other extreme is the excited schizo-affective patient who generally shows no residual defect other than his tendency toward episodes of recurrent illness. As a possible prophylactic measure, the excited schizo-affective patient can be maintained on a high-potency phenothiazine such as fluphenazine (Prolixin, Permitil), 2–10 mg daily, fluphenazine enanthate, or fluphenazine decanoate injections once every two weeks. Continued, intensive psychotherapy with the remitted, excited schizo-affective patient is not indicated and is usually rejected by the patient himself. However,

regular but infrequent contacts with the therapist are to be encouraged as a means of facilitating treatment should a psychotic
episode recur. At the time the patient is placed on long-term maintenance treatment, he and responsible family members should be
told of the need for prompt intervention should symptoms reappear.

Between the poor prognosis of the childhood asocial "process"
schizophrenic group and the good prognosis of the excited schizo-
affective group, are the retarded schizo-affective and the paranoid
groups. The recurrent, retarded schizo-affective patient may show
some residual signs of difficulty between episodes, including tendencies toward mystical thinking, inability to focus attention, loose
associations, self-isolatory trends, and increased eccentricity. Because these defects often become more pronounced after each
recurrence, it is recommended that such patients adhere to their
maintenance medication programs. This can frequently become a
major focus in counseling.

The paranoid patient typically exhibits significant residuals of his
illness after periods of psychotic exacerbation. These residuals may
include passivity and serious concerns about sexuality and potency.
A major dynamic seems to be the use of repressive mechanisms of
denial to exclude from awareness all internal difficulties and external pressures. Because of these patients' obvious psychological
conflicts concerning social and sexual roles, exploratory psychotherapy is frequently undertaken during the residual phase of their
illness. Antipsychotic medication should be used concurrently with
exploratory psychotherapy, for without such chemotherapeutic
support the added stress of psychotherapeutic interactions could
aggravate the patient's condition. Because of the social and sexual
inadequacy of many patients, particularly fearful paranoids, efforts
at social rehabilitation during the residual phase are potentially re-
warding. Even minimal heterosexual interaction, such as group
outings or dances, may provide sufficient social stimulation.

The goal of individual counseling with schizophrenic patients in
the residual stage is not the resolution of intrapsychic conflict, but
rather the provision of support, direction, and when necessary, help

in decision making. This must, of course, be done in a manner which does not rob the patient of the feeling of initiative and mastery, but rather in the spirit of cooperation in the resolution of problems of mutual concern.

OTHER INDICATIONS

Because the phenothiazines are so effective in treating the excited schizo-affective patient, it should come as no surprise to learn that these drugs also have marked mood-regularizing effects in acute manic states.

Manic States

The manic phase of manic-depressive illness is characterized by euphoric mood, giddiness, psychomotor excitation, flight of ideas, pressured speech, grandiose ideation, faulty judgment, and unjustified optimism. This is largely a reflection of the cyclic nature of this disorder, and manic patients improve in time.

Prior to the introduction of the phenothiazines, these manic cycles were unaffected by any therapeutic interventions. Now, dramatic, prompt reductions in symptomatology are seen when phenothiazines are used appropriately (high intramuscular doses initially, followed by chlorpromazine (Thorazine) 2000–3000 mg orally daily, or its equivalent, until symptomatic relief is obtained).

Excited patients have a great tolerance for phenothiazines. Positive effects can be expected whether the patient has had only recurrent manic episodes, or if he is either a manic-depressive patient in the manic phase, or an excited schizo-affective. When a significant feature of the total symptomatology is affective dysregulation of an excited, manic type, phenothiazines are definitely indicated.

Agitated Depression

As noted in Chapter 2, agitated depressions commonly occur in involutional patients, but are not necessarily restricted to that age group. The symptoms of agitated depression include a mixture of both manic and depressive features, and, in general, these patients respond well to phenothiazines, with a reduction or elimination in pacing, hand wringing, physical complaints, and a general amelioration of mood.

The overall therapeutic impact of either a tricyclic antidepressant or a phenothiazine in agitated depressions is *in general* about the same. A major difference, however, is the relative speed with which phenothiazines act to reduce psychomotor acceleration. Phenothiazines work quickly, while it may take two to three weeks before therapeutic effects emerge on antidepressant medication alone, and four to six weeks for maximum benefits. Consequently, some clinicians use a combination of these two drug classes, looking for an early effect from the phenothiazines and a synergistic (multiplicative) effect from combined treatment. This treatment strategy frequently allows for the reduction and ultimate withdrawal of the phenothiazine (which may have produced unwanted soporific effects) during the resolving stage of the patient's illness. The antidepressant can then be used for 6 months or so, in the range 50–150 mg imipramine (Tofranil) daily.

The Emotionally Unstable Personality

The mood-regularizing effects of the phenothiazines are of particular benefit in the treatment of the emotionally unstable personality (the closest APA diagnosis is 301.1, cyclothymic personality). Largely, but not exclusively adolescent females, these patients suffer serious mood swings over short time spans. Their moods may vary from giddy euphoria to depression with suicidal ideation, as often as several times during a single day. Significantly, these mood changes are not always related to environmental events, providing a clue that such patients may have faulty affect-regulating mechanisms. They seem unable to achieve emotional homeostasis, with a pattern of chronic overcorrection.

The phenothiazines almost always moderate the mood swings of the emotionally unstable personality (Klein and Davis, 1969). Typical therapeutic dose ranges are in the area 100–300 mg orally daily. Despite their good response to phenothiazines, emotionally unstable patients present particular psychotherapy and case mahagement problems because they generally do not regard mood stabilization in the same positive way as does the therapist. These patients seem "addicted" to their spontaneous "highs," and once their emotionality is leveled, their lives feel dull and uninteresting. Libido decrease or impaired sexual ability are possible drug side effects which can contribute to their feeling lifeless and empty. As a result, emotionally unstable patients are generally poorly motivated to continue with drug treatment. Maintaining these patients on prescribed medication can become a central (and frequently unsuccessful) focus in psychotherapy. Further complicating matters are the tendencies among these patients to a sensual life style, involving drug abuse and chaotic, promiscuous sexuality. Psychotherapy tends to be seen as square and stultifying.

On the positive side, follow-up of such patients (Rifkin *et al.*, 1972a) suggests that with maturation there is a trend toward normalization of the marked affective swings. By their early 30s, many formerly emotionally unstable patients have settled down, formed permanent interpersonal and heterosexual bonds, and are free of drug and alcohol abuse problems.

Contraindications

There are no established indications for antipsychotic agents in the treatment of neuroses, anxiety states, or retarded depressions.

The use of these agents, even in low doses, in hysterical patients is usually accompanied by increased symptomatology, particularly somatic complaints. Although these agents are widely used in the treatment of anticipatory and panic anxiety states, this is often inappropriate. While antidepressants and antianxiety agents are effective here, the utility of antipsychotics in neuroses and depression has not been established.

Side Effects

When the antipsychotic drugs are used in therapeutic doses, some side effects are likely. Many of these reactions, such as dry mouth, will be relatively minor, but a range of troublesome problems may develop, including blurred vision and dizziness. Other annoying problems, such as skin photosensitivity (where the skin burns deeply upon even minimal exposure to the sun) can usually be treated through preventive action. Side effects are considered fully in Chapter 8, but some major points are discussed here.

SOPORIFIC EFFECTS

Certain central nervous system effects (such as the sedative action of some phenothiazines) may be considered in some cases a side effect, and in other cases a principal therapeutic effect. For the manic patient exhausted from lack of sleep, a soporific phenothiazine would be the treatment of choice, since it is specific both for manic excitement and for the promotion of a more extended sleep pattern. When using this medication to induce more restful sleep, the skilled practitioner will prescribe the daily dosage to be taken an hour or two before bedtime, thereby taking advantage of the drug's sedative effect. Even when insomnia is not a problem, it is considered good practice to reduce daytime drowsiness by prescribing all or most of the drug at bedtime. Morning sleepiness induced by phenothiazines generally dissipates in time. Patients may have to be strenuously directed into activities, however, until the drowsiness wears off. There is no difference in the therapeutic effect of antipsychotic agents when given in equal, unequal, or once-daily doses.

EXTRAPYRAMIDAL SYNDROME (PARKINSONISM)

Most characteristic among the phenothiazine side effects is parkinsonism. Parkinsonism symptoms include a stiff, shuffling gait, tremor, lack of spontaneity and motor restlessness, fixed facial expression, and loss of associated movements (the free swing of torso and arms during walking). This rather dismal-sounding picture accounts for much of the "zombie" look frequently seen among patients at psychiatric hospitals (Hornykiewicz et al., 1970). The severity of such symptoms can generally be controlled, and in many cases eliminated entirely, through the appropriate use of anti-parkinson drugs, the most widely used of which are biperiden (Akineton), benztropine mesylate (Cogentin), procyclidine (Kemadrin), and trihexyphenidyl (Artane). However, antiparkinson agents themselves have occasionally been implicated in the development of schizophrenia-like symptoms, such as hallucinations. Often, after an initial period of antiparkinson drug treatment, this adjunctive medication can be safely withdrawn, without reappearance of parkinsonism.

DYSTONIC REACTIONS

Dystonic reactions are related to parkinsonism, producing uncontrolled, sometimes asymmetric, muscle activity, with stiffness or twisting of body parts. When pronounced, these reactions should be treated immediately with intramuscular administrations of antiparkinson agents or antihistamines.

TARDIVE DYSKINESIA

Dyskinesias involve disturbed, involuntary movements. One serious but rare reaction to chronic phenothiazine medication is *tardive dyskinesia*, usually consisting of uncontrolled, rhythmic, in-and-out ("fly-catching") movements of the tongue and throat, and rhythmic shaking or shuffling of the feet. This defect sometimes improves on withholding further drug treatment, but more often appears to be permanent and shows little or no response to antiparkinson drugs. Tardive dyskinesia is discussed more fully in Chapter 8.

CHAPTER **4**

ANTIANXIETY AGENTS AND SEDATIVES

Although the significant developments in modern psychopharmacology date from the early 1950s, a family of very widely used psychoactive drugs—the barbiturates—had been available for many years. These drugs were used not so much because of their efficacy, but rather because symptoms of anxiety were so ubiquitous an aspect of medical and psychiatric practice, and there were simply no other effective treatments available.

The barbiturates are central nervous system depressants, and in sufficient dosages can have a sedative effect. At lower doses, the effects are like those of alcohol, where suppression of higher cortical centers may have a mild euphoriant or depressant effect on mood, as well as adversely affecting psychomotor coordination. The barbiturates have the serious disadvantage of being addicting, so that increasing doses are usually required to produce similar psychological or behavioral effects. With habituation, the effective dose can approach very closely the lethal dose. Furthermore, with discontinuation, a former user will no longer be able to tolerate barbiturates at the same high level as when he was taking them regularly. Resumption of these drugs at formerly effective levels may be quite hazardous and accidental deaths among barbiturate users are not uncommon. Barbiturates also provide a painless, frequently used method of suicide.

Despite these shortcomings, prior to the 1950s, psychiatrists prescribed barbiturates widely, since there was little else available for quieting excited patients. A number of placebo-controlled comparative studies indicated that barbiturates do exhibit a modest superiority to placebo in calming neurotic and personality disorder patients (General Practitioner Research Group, 1964; Reynolds *et al.*, 1965; Wing and Lader, 1965).

The antianxiety agents (also known as minor tranquilizers or anxiolytics) were introduced into use in the late 1950s and early 1960s. There is little question that the magnitude of their therapeutic effects on anxiety is far greater than that of the barbiturates (Jenner *et al.*, 1961; Wheatley, 1968). Tables 4.1 and 4.2 enumerate the antianxiety agents, with representative dosage ranges given for the major members of these groups.

In addition to the barbiturates, other sedative and more potent hypnotic drugs now available include chloral hydrate (Noctec), paraldehyde (Paral), glutethimide (Doriden) and methyprylon (Noludar). The sedatives are listed in Table 4.3. The major drawbacks to these drugs are the extended drowsiness and poor motor coordination which they may produce. Also, they may be the cause of suicide, whether intended or accidental. As with the barbiturates, there is the possibility of addiction, with increasing doses necessary to maintain the same effects. Therefore, these sedative-hypnotic drugs seem to share all the negative features of barbiturates.

The relative therapeutic merits of the various antianxiety agents have been evaluated in a number of comparative studies. It would appear at this point, that in overall clinical effect there is relatively little difference among them (Ban, 1969; Rech and Moore, 1971).

In terms of drug management, compared to the propanediol (meprobamate) family of drugs (Miltown, Equanil, etc.) and the

TABLE 4.1. ANTIANXIETY AGENTS AND EFFECTIVE DOSAGE RANGES

Drug class	Generic name	Trade name(s)	Daily adult effective dose range (mg)		
			High	Moderate	Low
Benzodiazepines	Chlordiazepoxide	Librium	150–300	75–150	15–75
	Oxazepam	Serax	75–120	45–75	15–45
	Diazepam	Valium	24–40	16–24	4–16
Propanediols	Meprobamate	Equanil	1600–2400	1200–1600	800–1200
		Kesso-bamate			
		Miltown			
	Tybamate	Solacen	2000–3000	1250–2000	750–1250
Diphenylamines	Hydroxyzine	Atarax, Vistaril	200–400	100–200	50–100

TABLE 4.2. MISCELLANEOUS ANTIANXIETY AGENTS

Generic name	Trade name(s)	Manufacturer
Azacyclonol	Frenquel	Merrell
Benactyzine	Suavitil	Merck, Sharp & Dohme
Buclizine	Softran	Stuart
	Vibazine	Pfizer
Captodiame	Suvren	Ayerst
Chlormethazanone	Trancopal	Sterling-Winthrop
Ectylurea	Levanil	Upjohn
Hydroxyphenamate	Listica	Armour
Mephenoxalone	Lentran	Lakeside
	Trepidone	Lederle
Oxanamide	Quiactin	Merrell
Phenaglycodol	Ultran	Lilly

barbiturates, the benzodiazepines (Librium, Valium, Serax) are less depressing to the central nervous system vital centers and, therefore, more difficult to use for suicide. An additional advantage of the benzodiazepines over the barbiturates is that the difference between therapeutic and sedative doses is greater, allowing wider latitude in establishing optimal therapeutic dosages.

Anxiety reactions are usually self-limiting without drug intervention. However, certain patients may be intolerant of delay and demand immediate help. For such patients, particularly when there may be no clear antecedents for the anxiety, treatment with an antianxiety agent and brief, supportive psychotherapy or milieu manipulations may prove effective.

The issue of specific target areas for the various antianxiety agents has not yet been adequately studied. It is difficult to delineate specific indications for these drugs beyond the treatment of "anticipatory anxiety." Because anticipatory anxiety is an ubiquitous feature in obsessive, phobic, and depressed neurotics, antianxiety agents have found wide application in outpatient practice in general medicine, as well as in psychiatry.

TABLE 4.3. Sedatives (Barbiturate and Nonbarbiturate) and Hypnotics (Nonbarbiturate)

Generic name	Trade name(s)	Manufacturer
Barbiturate sedatives		
Amobarbital	Amytal	Lilly
Butabarbital	Butisol	McNeil
Heptabarbital	Medomin	Geigy
Mephobarbital	Mebaral	Winthrop
Metharbital	Gemonil	Abbott
Pentobarbital	Nembutal	Abbott
Phenobarbital	Eskabarb	Smith, Kline & French
	Luminal	Winthrop
	Stental	Robins
Secobarbital	Seconal	Lilly
Talbutal	Lotusate	Winthrop
Nonbarbiturate sedatives		
Acetylcarbromal	Sedamyl	Riker
Choral betaine	Beta-chlor	Mead Johnson
Chloral Hydrate	Felsules	Fellows Testagar
	Kessodrate	McKesson
	Noctec	Squibb
	Somnos	Merck, Sharp & Dohme
Paraldehyde	Paral	Fellows Testagar
Nonbarbiturate hypnotics		
Ethchlorvynol	Placidyl	Abbott
Ethinamate	Valmid	Lilly
Glutethimide	Doriden	Ciba
Methaqualone	Parest	Parke, Davis
	Quaalude	Royer
	Somnafac	Smith, Miller & Patch
	Sopor	Arnar-Stone
Methylpentynol	Dormison	Schering
Methyprylon	Noludar	Roche

Anticipatory Anxiety

Fears of specific objects or situations can be readily acquired through simple conditioning. The experimental acquisition of fear in animals has been demonstrated frequently in many species including man. Such fears provide powerful motivation for learning avoidance techniques to escape the anxiety-producing situation. While experimental animals may exhibit relatively normal behavior outside the laboratory in which their fears were acquired, man's special talent for long-range foresight makes him uniquely vulnerable to the development of chronic, anticipatory anxiety states.

A wide range of physical effects is associated with anticipatory anxiety, all of which may prove responsive to treatment with antianxiety agents. These effects include blushing in response to social threat or humiliation, disruptions in gastrointestinal and cardiac functioning in response to perceived physical threat, etc. Common concomitants of chronic anxiety states are muscular tension, headache, backache, and autonomic nervous system reactions such as dry mouth, sweating, pallor, and rapid heart rate.

Panic Anxiety

There is pharmacological evidence that *panic* anxiety may be psychophysiologically distinct from *anticipatory* anxiety. Autonomic signs may be more obvious and more intense, including sweating, dizziness, hot and cold flashes, diarrhea, vomiting, pounding, rapid heart beat, and fear of death. These dramatic symptoms, which are as intense as those experienced by individuals faced with imminent physical threat, can occur without any apparent precipitant.

It will be recalled from our earlier discussion of the antidepressant drugs that imipramine (Tofranil) and related agents have been found effective in treating the panic attacks of the separation-anxious patient (see Chapter 2). A common therapeutic error is the treatment of such patients with antianxiety agents (like Librium or Valium) alone. A therapeutic approach more in harmony with current evidence would encourage an initial trial of an antidepressant such as Tofranil in a phobic-anxious patient. Since this indication for the tricyclic antidepressants is not yet part of the working knowledge of most psychiatrists, requests for psychiatric consultation in such cases might be made with the suggestion to consider antidepressant medication. The patient with panic attacks is often treated ineffectively for long periods with sedatives, antianxiety agents, phenothiazines, or long-term intensive psychotherapy, without a trial of antidepressant medication being considered.

Dissociative and Conversion Reactions

Dissociative states (DSM-II diagnoses 300.14 and 300.6) refer to temporary disorganization of normal behavior patterns associated with altered states of consciousness. These include amnesias, fugue states, depersonalization, and sleepwalking.

Like dissociative states, conversion reactions are unusual behaviors which persist because of "secondary gains" derived by the patient (such as increased attention from others, lessened work responsibilities, etc.). These reactions typically take the form of somatic illness or functional impairment which fail to "make sense" medically (e.g., unexplainable paralysis of a limb). Signs of anxiety are usually absent, although clinical theoreticians frequently infer the presence of underlying anxiety states.

Generally, dissociative and conversion reactions are both refractory to drug treatment and should be handled psychotherapeutically. Even when anxiety is part of the symptom picture, the physician would do well to remember that hysterical patients often react negatively to almost any drug offered, including placebo, frequently with atypical side effects.

Phobic Reactions

It is characteristic of patients with specific phobias (DSM-II category 300.2) to exhibit high levels of associated anticipatory anxiety. This can frequently be ameliorated with the use of anti-anxiety agents. Phobias take many forms (Klein and Davis, 1969; Marks, 1969) but the most common classes include separation anxiety, fears of "aggressive" objects (such as knives, pins, etc.), fears of animals or insects, and fears of loss of control. The etiology of such disorders may be varied, and such speculations are beyond the scope of this book. However, it should be remembered that in addition to the acquisition of phobic behavior through conditioning, many species show innate responses which may interact with environmental events in complex ways. For example, cats show innate avoidance of "visual cliffs" without the "lesson" of having fallen over the edge; chicks and pups will pipe or whine for the absent mother without prior discomfort experiences of hunger or cold, etc.

In efforts at self-medication, phobic patients often abuse sedatives, alcohol, and stimulant drugs (Quitkin and Rifkin, 1972). The antianxiety agents, particularly the benzodiazepines, are a more suitable form of treatment. While these drugs may not completely eradicate anticipatory anxiety, they may reduce this to more endurable levels, with considerably greater physical and psychological safety.

Obsessive–Compulsive Reactions

Obsessive–compulsive patients (DSM-II category 300.3) characteristically experience repeated, unwanted, intrusive ideas or impulses to perform acts which are considered unreasonable. If prevented from performing these rituals, anxiety can be pronounced. Such patients seem to be refractory to all psychopharmacologic intervention. A few schizophrenic patients may present initially as severe obsessive–compulsives. In such cases a diagnostic-therapeutic trial of a phenothiazine may be indicated, with occasionally gratifying results.

However, the agitated depressive states frequently associated with these reactions may respond to either antidepressant or phenothiazine treatment, with concurrent lessening of obsessive–compulsive patterns.

Other Personality Disorders

Schizoid, passive–aggressive, emotionally unstable, and other personality disorders tend to be unresponsive to the minor tranquilizers. As noted in Chapter 3, emotionally unstable personalities will frequently respond positively to phenothiazines with mood leveling; antianxiety agents do not seem to be indicated.

Sleep Problems

Sleep problems such as insomnia, inability to remain asleep, early morning awakening, bad dreams, nightmares, sleep talking, and sleepwalking, are nonspecific concomitants of many psychiatric disorders. For many years physicians have prescribed sedative drugs to help patients fall asleep and remain asleep. Barbiturates can be quite helpful for these target symptoms, but the risk of habituation, abuse, and toxicity are relatively high. These dangers are insignificant with the benzodiazepines (such as Valium), and increasingly such drugs are being prescribed to be taken upon retiring when sleep difficulties are the principal target.

CHAPTER 5

LITHIUM

Studies in Australia prior to 1950 indicated the probable utility of the element lithium for treating manic patients; however, it was not until about 1965 that this drug came into more general use. European psychiatrists began paying serious attention to lithium as an anti-manic agent in the late 1950s, and a number of controlled, evaluative studies appeared in the 1960s (Johnson *et al.*, 1968; Maggs, 1963; Schou, 1968). This effort is continuing with large-scale, on-going, cooperative studies involving the National Institute of Mental Health and the Veterans Administration. The weight of clinical and experimental evidence makes it clear that lithium is an effective treatment for manic states (Gattozzi, 1970).

The delay between discovery and introduction of lithium into clinical practice in this country provides an interesting aside, il-lustrating some of the problems of scientific communication, as well as the hazards of placing drug development and promulgation in the hands of companies whose principal concern is for profits and losses.

Part of the difficulty in spreading the word about lithium was the professional and geographic isolation of Australia, the place of its discovery. In addition, in the late 1940s and early 1950s, psychiatrists were not attuned to pharmacology; thus even if communication had been better, these findings might still have fallen on deaf ears. Also, the toxic hazards of lithium are certainly greater than with many other psychotropic drugs, and this tended to discourage its use. In the 1940s, indiscriminate use of lithium as a salt substitute for cardiac patients resulted in a number of well-publicized fatalities. A further consideration was the fact that as a diagnostic group, manic patients are relatively rare and tend not to be a principal therapeutic concern for most mental health practitioners. Probably most important in impeding the development of lithium for general use was the fact that its low cost and ready availability made it unprofitable for private drug company development. Lithium could be obtained, commercially packaged in 50 and 100 lb. sacks for industrial use, for just a few dollars. Therefore, the drug companies had no profit incentive for supporting clinical trials, as is customary in new drug research. It was only in the late 1960s that several United States' companies, responding to pressure from American psychiatrists, decided to make lithium available as a pharmaceutical.

Manic States

Therapeutic doses of lithium for acute mania are usually in the range 1500–2500 mg daily. Ordinarily, lithium (prepared in 300 mg tablets) is started at about 600–900 mg on the first day, reaching 1200–1800 mg on the second day. Adjustments thereafter are made according to the patient's clinical condition and are monitored principally according to blood lithium levels. These should range between 1.0 and 2.0 mEq/liter per day. Serum (blood) levels below 1.0 are rarely effective therapeutically (except in older patients), while levels in excess of 2.0 almost certainly lead to toxic manifestations.

Due to individual differences in physiology, the usual therapeutic guide of milligrams of drug/kilograms of body weight is too crude. To ensure adequate dose levels, in the initial stages of lithium treatment, blood tests should be done once or twice a week. Blood lithium levels should not exceed 2.0 mEq/liter. When maintenance dosage levels have been determined, blood testing can be reduced in frequency, but should be done every other month once dosage has been stabilized. Customarily, the physician will attempt to maintain blood lithium levels at between .8 and 1.5 mEq/liter, a nontoxic, generally therapeutic blood level.

Other therapies for acute manic states include the soporific phenothiazines such as chlorpromazine (Thorazine), or butyrophenones such as haloperidol (Haldol). ECT has been tried but is unpopular because of generally low-level effectiveness, high relapse rate, induced organic mental syndromes, and poor patient acceptance.

The antipsychotic agents control manic states with pronounced sedative effects, but Schou (1968) feels that the underlying symptoms of mania (elevated mood, flight of ideas, distractability) are unaffected by these drugs. According to his theory, manic behavior is "contained" by antipsychotic agents until the manic episode remits, while lithium attacks manic symptomatology at all levels, without sedation. However, for acute treatment, lithium's speed of action is somewhat slow, with full effects not evident for 5–10 days or more. In addition, recent evidence (Prien et al., 1972a) indicates that lithium is less effective than chlorpromazine in treating the highly active, acute manic patient. Thus, the most efficient treatment of an acute manic patient would involve the simultaneous use of an antipsychotic agent (either a phenothiazine or butyrophenone) in high dosages and lithium. The antipsychotic agent will usually produce a rapid effect and then can be phased out within several weeks, with long-term maintenance on lithium alone.

Interested readers are referred to articles by Prien et al. (1970, 1971, 1972a,b), Schou (1968), and the National Institute of Mental Health (Gattozzi, 1970) which support the utility of lithium in the treatment of acute manic states.

Because of the toxic risk, patients (and those in positions of responsibility for the patient) must be impressed with the necessity for taking *exactly* the prescribed number of capsules at the *time* they are prescribed. The dosage range for lithium is much more limited than for other psychoactive drugs. Lithium is never to be used on an "as needed" basis. However, it should be understood that when the drug is properly monitored and taken as prescribed, the risk of serious side effects is low.

Other Indications

Because the introduction of lithium into psychiatric practice has been relatively recent, other indications for the drug, beyond acute manic states, are not clearly established. It is possible that in some cases of psychomotor excitement related either to catatonic schizophrenic states or schizo-affective psychoses, lithium may prove to be an effective calming agent (Schlagenhauf *et al.*, 1966). It would not be unusual for a psychiatrist who found phenothiazines ineffective in relieving an excited patient to use lithium as a potentially effective calming agent. Other exploratory uses of lithium include the treatment of premenstrual tension (Sletten and Gershon, 1966), mood disorders in children (Annell, 1969) and young adults (Rifkin *et al.*, 1972b), and the treatment of patients with explosive behavior outbursts. While clinically suggestive, the supporting evidence for the efficacy of lithium in these other states is not yet available (Gershon and Shopsin, 1972).

Evidence on the long-term effects of lithium on relapse rates and the issue of preventive treatment are discussed in Chapter 9. It can be stated here, however, that many manic-depressive patients should be maintained on lithium for prophylactic purposes, and this in itself may raise certain psychotherapeutic or counseling problems —often threats of jail, hospitalization, and divorce have to be made to force manic patients into taking their medicine. It is difficult to encourage patients who are feeling well to continue on medication. A significant management problem with the recurrent manic patient is that when euphoric, his high spirits make it almost impossible for him to understand that he is suffering from a cyclic disorder requiring prompt, active treatment. This point usually has to be hammered home repeatedly during the post-manic recovery period when the patient may be more willing to acknowledge his debt to psychopharmacologic treatment. It may be particularly hard to make this point with a patient who has had only one manic episode. However, unless the family is particularly tolerant and alert to early signs of difficulty, the *probable* recurrent nature of the disorder speaks strongly for prophylactic lithium treatment.

Contraindications

Because of the side effect risks associated with lithium, the use of this drug in routine practice should be restricted to disorders for which indications are established. At present this means acute treatment of manic or excited states and prophylactic use in manic-depressive illness. However, as the research evidence accumulates, these indications may be broadened.

Side Effects

The side effect of lithium which most concerns the practitioner is death. However, there is a progression of lithium-related side effects (See Chapter 8) which provide ample warning that dosage levels should be reduced. It is not unusual for some patients to exhibit a fine hand tremor which is unresponsive to antiparkinson drug treatment. Gastrointestinal disturbances are frequent during the early stages of treatment. They take the form of diarrhea, nausea, anorexia, vomiting or abdominal pain, and can usually be dealt with by temporarily reducing dosage until the patient adapts, after which the dosage can generally be increased successfully. Other, more serious toxic reactions involve such neurological symptoms as muscular weakness, tremor, difficulty walking, impaired movements, sleepiness, difficulty talking, dizziness, blurred vision, and possible seizures or coma. There have also been reports of thyroid dysfunction concomitant with lithium use.

To ensure proper cell metabolism, normal salt intake is necessary. Usually this simply means following a regular diet: patients on salt-free diets should not take lithium. In addition, patients may need to be encouraged to eat properly, since lithium may cause a temporary loss of appetite. Lithium may precipitate thyroid deficiency, which often manifests itself by fatigue, dry skin, and sensitivity to cold.

Obviously, while lithium is not an innocuous drug, it is quite effective for its target populations. Yet even when lithium is being carefully administered, the nonmedical practitioner has a responsibility to monitor possible central nervous system side effects, the occurrence of which should be *immediately* related to the treating physician.

CHAPTER 6

STIMULANTS

Stimulants are widely used in general medicine, particularly as appetite depressants, but they have little place in modern psychopharmacologic practice. A major exception to this concerns the drug treatment of hyperactive children, discussed later in this chapter. Members of the stimulant drug category are listed in Table 6.1; they include the widely used (and abused) amphetamines, as well as deanol and methylphenidate.

In normal individuals, the stimulants can produce a sense of well-being, competence, or mild euphoria, and are associated with feelings of decreased need for food and sleep. Stimulants are widely used by students studying for examinations, by long haul truck drivers, and others seeking to increase endurance. With extended use, tenseness and irritability are common. There is some evidence to support the belief of improved psychomotor performance during acute amphetamine use (Holliday, 1965). Consequently, these drugs are a favorite of athletes engaged in tests of endurance such as track meets and long-distance bicycle races.

There has been growing sophistication among drug abusers about the hazards of extended stimulant use (embodied in the frequent

TABLE 6.1. Stimulant Drugs

Generic name	Trade name	Manufacturer
	Amphetamines	
Amphetamine	Benzadrine	Smith, Kline & French
Benzphetamine	Didrex	Upjohn
Dextroamphetamine	Dexedrine	Smith, Kline & French
	Dexa-Sequels	Lederle
	Dexa-Span	USV Pharmaceutical
	Obotan	Mallinckrodt
	PERKёONE	Ascher
Levoamphetamine	Amodril	North American
	Cydril	Tutag
	Pedestal	Len-Tag
Methamphetamine	Amphedroxyn	Lilly
	Desoxyn	Abbott
	Methedrine	Burroughs-Wellcome
	Nonamphetamines	
Deanol	Deaner	Riker
Methylphenidate	Ritalin	Ciba
Pentylenetetrazol	Metrazol	Knoll
	Nioric	Ascher
Phenmetrazine	Preludin	Geigy

warning, "Speed kills"). The need for caution in the use of stimulants is indisputable. Being "spaced-out" on amphetamines is a well-known phenomenon referring to a lack of physical and psychological responsiveness. Instead of being alert and "up," the "spaced-out" drug abuser is socially unresponsive, attentive only to his own thoughts, and frequently unable to communicate intelligently; semi-starved, he has no desire to eat; exhausted, he is unable to sleep. Rounding out this rather dismal picture, decreased sexual ability or complete loss of sexual competence is common. Since amphetamine abusers frequently abuse barbiturates also, it is difficult to isolate the unique effects of each drug.

In addition, amphetamine psychoses are a real possibility. These are usually flagrantly paranoid states which, although reversible, do not dissipate immediately upon discontinuation of the drug. Other manifestations of a toxic psychosis such as confusion and disorientation may be present, and may include visual hallucinations (Kalant, 1966).

Reactive Depressions

About the only possible psychiatric indication for stimulants in adults is for clearly reactive depressions in individuals with no prior history of psychological difficulty (Klein and Davis, 1969). In the case of patients with prior emotional instability or psychotic episodes, the use of stimulants is clearly contraindicated because of the possibility of precipitating further instability. Stimulant use must be carefully monitored, since drug tolerance may develop quickly, requiring increased dosage to maintain positive mood effects, while running the risk of producing other unwanted effects.

To reiterate, these drugs should be used only rarely. On the few occasions when they are used therapeutically, it should be for the short-term only. Extended use (beyond 6–8 weeks) should be seriously questioned. Certain stimulants, however, are indicated in the treatment of hyperactive children.

The Hyperactive (Hyperkinetic) Child

Increasing attention is being paid to the field of child psychopharmacology, notably treatment of the hyperactive child. Such preadolescent children, with a sex ratio of approximately four boys to one girl, present particular problems to the school and to their families. While usually of normal intelligence or better, these children may have a history of repeated school failure, with reports of poor study habits, distractibility, uncooperativeness, and disruptiveness in school and at home. These highly distractible children have particular difficulty working toward long-range goals. Their constant motor activity disturbs other children, as well as preventing the child himself from sitting still long enough to learn what is being taught. Some studies indicate that the hyperactive child's *total* motor output may not differ significantly from that of a normal child; instead, their problem may relate to rather persistent motor behavior. Normal children seem to be able to remain calm and attentive for long periods, with high energy bursts of motor activity reserved for socially sanctioned opportunities such as recess or play periods.

Hyperactive children are frequently friendly, with considerable personal charm, but seem unable to exercise the behavioral controls expected by adults. Since with maturation much of the hyperactivity is outgrown, this phenomenon likely reflects a developmental lag. The problem can be conceptualized as the failure of the developing cerebral cortex to exert the necessary inhibitory control over the activity of other brain centers. Stimulant drugs presumably make the cerebral cortex temporarily more efficient, so it can exert greater inhibitory control over the activity of lower brain centers.

Studies by Conners (1969) and others indicate that the hyperactive, distractible child under age 12, can generally be helped toward a more satisfactory adjustment and more acceptable school performance through long-term use of stimulants.

Geriatric Psychiatry

Many geriatric patients are sluggish and apathetic. There is some evidence that stimulants such as pentylenetetrazol (Metrazol) may have a positive effect on relieving apathy in geriatric patients (Lifschitz and Kline, 1970). There is also some evidence (Chien, 1971) indicating that beer may serve as an antiapathy agent for geriatric groups. If this finding is substantiated, beer would seem to be a desirable agent, in part because it could promote increased socialization, since most people tend to prefer drinking in groups rather than alone. Secondarily, it could be a useful nutritional supplement. Stimulants have a depressing effect on appetite, clearly undesirable in elderly patients, many of whom may have a problem maintaining adequate body weight and nutrition.

Since stimulants can also exacerbate an incipient psychosis, and the probability of toxic psychosis is greater in patients with suspected cerebral defect, stimulants should be avoided in the elderly, or used very discretely.

Side Effects

We have already considered some of the negative effects of nonprescribed stimulant use. Other possible unwanted effects include:

1. Heart palpitations (pounding heart)
2. Tachycardia (rapid heart rate)
3. Elevated blood pressure
4. Insomnia
5. Tremor
6. Headache
7. Dry mouth
8. Bad taste in mouth
9. Diarrhea
10. Anorexia (loss of appetite)

CHAPTER 7

ELECTROCONVULSIVE TREATMENT (ECT)

While a discussion of electroconvulsive treatment may not seem relevant in a volume on drug therapy, ECT is, nevertheless, a widely used and effective somatic treatment, prescribed both independently and in combination with psychotropic drugs.

In the standard form of ECT treatment, a brief electrical current is passed between two electrodes placed at the patient's temples. The voltage, amperage, and duration of the current are under the control of the physician, and the treatment is generally administered in sufficient strength to render the patient unconscious and produce a grand mal seizure. To control the gross muscular contractions and reduce the hazards of bone fracture, most practitioners use muscle relaxants (such as succinylcholine) shortly before the ECT treatment. Many therapists also use a short-acting anesthesia to put the patient to sleep just prior to the treatment.

As a general guide to practice, the number of ECT treatments administered in depressives is usually dictated by symptomatic relief. In schizophrenia, most practitioners feel that a complete "course" of 14–20 treatments is necessary to prevent immediate relapse. Typically, ECT produces amnesia and a temporary post-seizure confusional state which may persist for days or perhaps weeks during which the patient may exhibit impaired verbal ability and disorientation.

ECT was widely practiced in the years 1933–1955. During this period patients did not have the benefit of muscle relaxants or anes-thetics preliminary to ECT treatments, and many suffered great apprehensiveness anticipating the treatment-induced loss of mental and muscular control. Perhaps in response to the excesses of that period, along with poor acceptance by patients, use of this treat-ment form has declined markedly.

As interest grew in the sociology of the psychiatric hospital, workers in all mental health disciplines denigrated ECT further, suspecting it of being used punitively, rather than therapeutically. Consequently, since 1955 there has been a turning away from ECT with a tendency to stereotype it as a primitive and brutal form of treatment, the use of which, if encouraged, leads to abuse. However, such dangers are inherent in any form of psychiatric or psycho-logical treatment. We all know of practitioners who have abused the psychotherapeutic relationship. Since it is possible to abuse any therapeutic medium, to foreclose one's treatment planning because of this possibility is both scientifically and professionally unsound. It is the responsibility of each mental health worker to become as familiar as possible with the indications and contraindications for all forms of treatment and, when necessary, to refer to responsible practitioners. Many organically oriented psychiatrists use ECT in a responsible manner, particularly when treating retarded or agitated depressives, or patients with catatonic schizophrenia.

Comparative studies of ECT and antidepressant drugs indicate that ECT is at least as successful as the antidepressant drugs in regularly producing good-to-excellent, short-term effects in depres-sed patients (Greenblatt et al., 1962, 1964; Robin and Harris, 1962).

However, ECT has its disadvantages. Both naturally occurring seizures and electrically induced convulsions produce a reversible organic mental syndrome—a condition of confused thinking, forgetfulness, and disorientation. Beyond the period of the immediate post-ECT confusional state, most standard psychological tests show little or no cognitive impairment. For most patients there appears clinically to be a return to normal functioning within a month or two after the last ECT treatment. It has not been clearly established that the postseizure organic mental syndrome is associated with permanent brain damage, but clinical experience suggests that patients subjected to repeated courses of ECT often exhibit loss of intellectual capability, have difficulty in new learning, and develop abnormally rigid personalities. All of this suggests that permanent brain damage is possible with repeated ECT use. However, a refinement in ECT technique may reduce the possibility. Initial studies indicate that *unilateral* ECT, applied to the nondominant hemisphere, (i.e., the side of brain *not* principally involved with speech mechanisms) is therapeutically equivalent to the standard *bilateral* procedure, while producing a much less pronounced organic mental syndrome (Bidder *et al.*, 1970; Cohen *et al.*, 1968; Cannicott *et al.*, 1967; Strain *et al.*, 1968).

The drawbacks to ECT are somewhat offset by its potentially more rapid speed of action (compared to the 2–4 weeks required for most antidepressant drugs). Therefore, a therapeutic dilemma frequently faced by the psychiatrist is a choice between slower-acting antidepressant drugs and ECT. If antidepressant drugs are chosen as the sole therapeutic route, an additional month or more of treatment must be carefully evaluated by the psychiatrist, considering the possible suicidal risk in many depressed individuals. If there is reason to doubt the ability of responsible family members or hospital staff to adequately monitor a patient with significant suicidal risk, a prompt decision to use ECT is probably entirely justified. In weighing these treatment alternatives, the physician must also consider the physical status of the patient. This is particularly true of older patients who may have cardiac abnormalities.

Surprisingly, the incidence of cardiac arrest during ECT is very low and most enlightened practitioners consider the hazards of anti-depressant drug therapy in older patients with heart conditions greater than the hazards of ECT. The lowered blood pressure caused by some antidepressant drugs may pose a severe risk of falls, with associated fractures.

Because of ECT's side effects, however, as a general treatment strategy it is usually preferable to treat most depressed patients initially with antidepressant drugs. Most patients are neither so suicidal nor so depressed that they require immediate ECT. With sufficient surveillance, many depressed patients can be managed safely either at home or in the hospital, using antidepressant drug treatment alone. If, after 4 weeks on adequate doses of one of the tricyclic drugs (such as Tofranil or Elavil) an adequate response has not been obtained, then an MAO inhibitor could be tried, while holding ECT as a fallback treatment strategy. If the patient proves unresponsive to both drug trials, then ECT should be seriously considered.

Side Effects

As noted earlier ECT carries with it the side effects of a post-seizure, acute organic mental syndrome with amnesia, confusion, and recent memory loss. After long, repeated courses of ECT there may be difficulty in learning new material and sometimes there is the development of a rigid personality.

Convulsive therapy is also associated with a risk of occasional vertebral or long bone fractures. Through the use of muscle relax-ants just before the application of the convulsive shock, these hazards can usually be avoided. However, use of such muscle relaxants as succinylcholine (frequently in conjunction with a short-acting anesthetic drug) has certain inherent risks. These drugs temporarily suppress respiration so that an anesthesiologist must be available to do artificial pulmonary ventilation. In addition, suppression of breathing by muscle relaxants, if there has been no prior sedation, is associated psychologically with an overwhelming panicky feeling of impending doom. Fortunately, the subsequent electrical treatment produces amnesia in many patients, so that this disturbing experience may not be recalled.

Rationale for ECT:
1 - high suicide risk +
hence can't wait for TCA
to take effect (10 day - 3 wks)

2. Elderly ptnts w/ heart
probs.

3 - Refractory of TCA & MAOI

CHAPTER **8**

SIDE EFFECTS

Some major side effects of the various psychotropic drugs have been discussed in Chapters 2–6. This chapter provides additional information on the side-effects characteristic of the major drug classes.

Sensitivity to reports of side effects is essential to the patient's welfare. In collaborating with a psychiatrist, the nonmedical practitioner will often have more frequent contact with a patient. The information in this chapter is designed to provide the necessary background information to evaluate a patient's reports of side effects.

All active drugs can produce unwanted effects. The basic mechanisms for controlling or eliminating these are:

1. Dosage reduction
2. Drug discontinuation
3. Drug change
4. Adjunctive medication

For some relatively mild side effects, no special steps are necessary since such effects are usually expected to dissipate as the body accommodates to the drug. Thus, mild effects, such as dry mouth, which often accompany the introduction of a new psychoactive drug, can generally be ignored with the expectation that the reaction will soon disappear. Other effects like orthostatic hypotension (feeling dizzy and light-headed upon standing up) are usually well tolerated by patients, as long as they are given some reassurances. In the case of nonserious side effects, the physician will have to evaluate the potential benefits to be derived from continued treatment versus the patient's discomfort. Frequently, temporary dosage reduction eliminates side effects, after which the drug can be increased without distress. However, the patient (and his therapist) is not always so lucky, so that at times a choice has to be made between changing the drug, discontinuing the drug completely, reducing dosage permanently, or using adjunctive medication to relieve side effects.

Only occasionally will drugs have to be discontinued completely. Certain rare reactions involving blood, liver, or cardiac abnormalities may be life-threatening, and psychotropic drugs must be discontinued until the medical risk has passed. After successful medical treatment, medication, possibly with another class of psychotropic drug, can be reinstituted. Control of most side effects is usually possible, however, through methods other than drug discontinuation.

In evaluating a patient's side effects reports, one must bear in mind that what is perceived by the patient as a side effect may well be a symptom of his psychiatric disorder. Depressed patients frequently report problems of constipation, anorexia, loss of sexual ability, or vague pains. The somatic delusions of schizophrenics can also be reported as drug reactions. Conversely, some unwanted drug effects can readily be mistaken for psychopathological symptoms. For example, phenothiazines frequently induce psychomotor slowing which is easily misinterpreted as symptomatic of depression. Imipramine (Tofranil) can induce patterned visual images which can be misevaluated as spontaneous hallucinatory experiences. Therefore, knowing some of the expected side reactions of the various drugs in common use will aid in evaluating the credibility of a patient's reports. However, without good individual base-rate data, it is often difficult to distinguish between symptom and side effect.

The following is a general overview of some of the major types of side effects observed in patients receiving psychotropic drugs. Specific information on the various drug classes appears later.

Central Nervous System Effects

Most prominent among the CNS side effects are the extrapyramidal effects, including parkinsonism, dystonia, dyskinesia, and akathisia.

THE PARKINSON SYNDROME

This constellation of symptoms includes muscular rigidity, tremor, postural alterations, and notably akinesia (decrease in spontaneous movements). Quite commonly associated with these are a fixed, masklike facial expression, shuffling gait, drooling, and loss of associated movements (free swing of arms when walking).

DYSTONIA

Uncoordinated, spasmodic movements of the body and limbs.

DYSKINESIA

Involuntary, coordinated, repetitive, stereotyped movements.

Akathisia

Involuntary motor restlessness, inability to sit still, and constant fidgeting.

These CNS side effects are produced by all classes of antipsychotic drugs: the phenothiazines, butyrophenones, and thioxanthenes. Such reactions will tend to appear within the first month or so of phenothiazine treatment. The dystonias and dyskinesias can develop within 1 hour of the first administration (much to the dismay of the patient, family, and doctor). Some of these effects are quite dramatic. Most psychiatrists are familiar with the milder manifestations of parkinsonism and handle the situation with dosage modification or oral antiparkinson medication. However, a severe dystonia, where the patient's head and neck are contorted and swallowing is difficult, requires immediate emergency attention, usually in the form of intramuscular or intravenous antiparkinson agents. Relief should be immediate.

Drowsiness

This is a common side effect with all psychotropic medication, although chlorpromazine (Thorazine) and thioridazine (Mellaril) may produce more sedation than some other drugs. Many patients, with no change in dosage regimen, develop a tolerance to this effect within several weeks of treatment.

Autonomic Nervous System Effects

An extensive catalog of annoying autonomic effects has been observed in patients receiving psychotropic drugs. These effects include:

1. Blurred vision
2. Constipation
3. Diarrhea
4. Dizziness
5. Dry mouth
6. Ejaculation disturbance or inhibition
7. Faintness
8. Galactorrhea (discharge from the nipple in males or females)
9. Gynecomastia (breast growth)
10. Menstrual changes
11. Nasal congestion
12. Nausea
13. Orthostatic hypotension (dizziness or "black-out" upon rising quickly)
14. Urinary difficulty (slow starting stream)

Rare Side Effects

AGRANULOCYTOSIS

Agranulocytosis is a serious blood abnormality in which a patient's normal white blood count drops precipitously; this condition is usually associated with high fever and throat infection. Emergency medical attention is essential. There is a serious risk of death, in part because of the patient's lessened resistance to infection. If the patient survives the first day or two, recovery is usually rapid (7–10 days).

HEPATITIS

Abnormalities of liver function are occasionally reported due to psychotropic drugs. This can be serious, but the patient usually responds to drug discontinuation or change. The most obvious symptom is a jaundiced appearance, usually preceded by fever, general malaise, and gastrointestinal disturbances.

TARDIVE DYSKINESIA

This rare, treatment-resistant form of dyskinesia can occur after years of psychotropic treatment, sometimes after discontinuation of phenothiazines, but also during short-term phenothiazine use. The syndrome includes uncontrollable sucking or smacking lip movements, and forward and backward tongue movements; swallowing may also be difficult. Uncontrolled movements of the hands or feet may be observed as well, although the head and neck are principally affected. Tardive dyskinesia remains untreatable and does not usually remit spontaneously.

Side Effects of the Major Drug Classes

Tables 8.1–8.6 provide, in tabular form, a convenient summary of the relative incidence of side effects in 10 phenothiazines and 6 antidepressants. These tables (adapted from Klein and Davis, 1969) are based on published reports of many investigators, and because of variations in study method the incidences reported can be considered only approximate. In these tables the following conventions were followed:

very frequent: observed in 20% or more of patients treated;
frequent: 10–20% observed incidence;
occasional: 5–10%;
rare: 1–5%;
very rare: less than 1%.

Further detail on side effects specific to certain drug classes follows.

TABLE 8.1. Central Nervous System Side Effects of 10 Phenothiazines[a]

Generic name	Extrapyramidal	Dystonia	Akathisia	Seizures	Drowsiness	Confusion	Depression
Acetophenazine	Frequent	Rare	Rare	Rare	Occasional	?	?
Chlorpromazine	Frequent	Rare	Frequent	Rare	Very frequent	Occasional	Frequent
Fluphenazine	Frequent	Occasional	Frequent	Very rare	Frequent	?	?
Mepazine	Rare	Rare	Frequent	Very rare	Very frequent	?	Occasional
Perphenazine	Very frequent	Rare	Very frequent	Very rare	Frequent	?	Occasional
Prochlorperazine	Very frequent	Rare	Occasional	Very rare	Occasional	?	Rare
Promazine	Very frequent	?	?	Frequent	Occasional	Frequent	?
Thioridazine	Occasional	Rare	Occasional	Rare	Very frequent	Occasional	Very rare
Trifluoperazine	Very frequent	Rare	Rare	Rare	Very frequent	?	Rare
Triflupromazine	Occasional	Rare	Occasional	Very rare	Frequent	?	Rare

[a]After Klein and Davis (1969).

TABLE 8.2. Autonomic Nervous System Side Effects of 10 Phenothiazines[a]

Generic name	Dizziness	Dry mouth	Disturbed sexual function	Urinary disturbance	Nasal stuffiness	Visual disturbance	Hypotension	Constipation	Diarrhea
Acetophenazine	Frequent	?	?	?	?	Rare	Rare	?	?
Chlorpromazine	Occasional	Very frequent	?	Rare	Rare	Frequent	Rare	Frequent	Very rare
Fluphenazine	Occasional	Occasional	?	Very rare	Occasional	Rare	Very rare	Occasional	Very rare
Mepazine	Frequent	Very frequent	?	?	?	Very frequent	?	Very frequent	?
Perphenazine	Occasional	Frequent	?	?	Very rare	Frequent	Very rare	Rare	?
Prochlorperazine	Occasional	Frequent	?	?	Very frequent	Frequent	?	Rare	?
Promazine	Occasional	Occasional	?	?	?	?	Frequent	?	?
Thioridazine	Very frequent	Very frequent	?	Occasional	?	Frequent	Rare	Frequent	Rare
Trifluoperazine	Very frequent	Rare	Rare	Very rare	?	Rare	Very rare	Very rare	Very rare
Triflupromazine	Frequent	Occasional	?	Very rare	Rare	Occasional	?	Rare	Very rare

[a] After Klein and Davis (1969).

TABLE 8.3. MISCELLANEOUS SIDE EFFECTS OF 10 PHENOTHIAZINES[a]

Generic name	Allergic reactions	Anorexia	Blood disturbance	Endocrine effects	Liver abnormality	Nausea, vomiting	Weight change
Acetophenazine	Rare	?	?	Rare	?	?	?
Chlorpromazine	Occasional	Rare	Very rare	Occasional	Rare	Rare	Very frequent
Fluphenazine	Rare	?	?	Rare	Very rare	Rare	?
Mepazine	Rare	?	?	?	?	Rare	?
Perphenazine	Very rare	Rare	?	Very rare	Very rare	Rare	Occasional
Prochlorperazine	Rare	Frequent	?	Rare	Very rare	Rare	Frequent
Promazine	?	?	?	?	?	Rare	?
Thioridazine	Rare	Very rare	Rare	Rare	Very rare	Very frequent	?
Trifluoperazine	Rare	Frequent	Rare	Very rare	Rare	Rare	Very rare
Triflupromazine	Rare	Very rare	?	Very rare	Very rare	Rare	Rare

[a] After Klein and Davis (1969).

72

TABLE 8.4. Central Nervous System Side Effects of Six Major Antidepressants[a]

Generic name	Confusion	Drowsiness	Hyperactivity	Tremor
Tricyclics				
Amitriptyline	Rare	Frequent	Occasional	Frequent
Imipramine	Rare	Frequent	Occasional	Frequent
Inhibitors				
Isocarboxazid	Rare	Occasional	Frequent	Occasional
Nortriptyline	Rare	Occasional	Occasional	Rare
Phenelzine	Rare	Occasional	Frequent	Occasional
Tranylcypromine	?	Rare	?	?

[a] After Klein and Davis (1969).

Phenothiazines

In addition to the material considered in Chapter 3, several additional topics warrant attention (see Table 8.7).

Skin and Eye Changes

Photosensitivity Some patients on phenothiazines, particularly chlorpromazine, may show a marked sensitivity to sunlight, developing a serious sunburn quite readily. Thus, patients taking phenothiazines should avoid exposure to the sun by wearing protective clothing, large sun hats, or by coating the skin with sunscreening lotions. An infrequent reaction associated with long-term phenothiazine use is skin discoloration, starting as a deep tan and progressing through slate gray to a bluish-purple.

Lens and Retina Effects Long term use of high dosages of phenothiazines, particularly chlorpromazine (Thorazine) and thioridazine (Mellaril), may lead to the development of opaque spots in the

TABLE 8.5. Autonomic Nervous System Side Effects of Six Major Antidepressants[a]

Generic name	Constipation	Dizziness	Dry mouth	Libido decrease	Libido increase	Sweating	Urinary retention	Visual disturbance
Tricyclics								
Amitriptyline	Frequent	Very frequent	Very frequent	Rare	Occasional	Very frequent	Occasional	Frequent
Imipramine	Frequent	Very frequent	Very frequent	Rare	Occasional	Very frequent	Occasional	Frequent
MAO Inhibitors								
Isocarboxazid	Occasional	Frequent	Frequent	Rare	Occasional	Frequent	Occasional	Frequent
Nortriptyline	Rare	Occasional	Frequent	?	?	Rare	?	Rare
Phenelzine	Occasional	Frequent	Very frequent	Rare	Occasional	Frequent	Occasional	Frequent
Tranylcypromine	Rare	Occasional	Occasional	?	?	?	?	Occasional

[a]After Klein and Davis (1969).

74

TABLE 8.6. Miscellaneous Side Effects of Six Major Antidepressants[a]

Generic Name	Nausea	Palpitation	Edema
Tricyclics			
Amitriptyline	Occasional	Occasional	Very rare
Imipramine	Occasional	Occasional	Very rare
MAO Inhibitors			
Isocarboxazid	Occasional	Rare	Occasional
Nortriptyline	Rare	?	?
Phenelzine	Occasional	Rare	Occasional
Tranylcypromine	Rare	Rare	?

[a]After Klein and Davis (1969).

cornea or lens, or retinal changes. These changes are usually of no functional consequence and are observable only in ophthalmic examination. However, if these changes are severe, some visual impairment is possible. The tendency to develop eye changes appears to be greater in patients with skin discoloration than in those not so affected. However, these changes tend to be slowly reversible, so that after switching to another phenothiazine, the eye normalizes within 6 months to 1 year.

Butyrophenones

Although unrelated chemically to the phenothiazines, the butyrophenones have similar clinical effects and side effects. These drugs have not been as widely studied as the phenothiazines, so less detail is available on the relative incidence of specific side effects. Butyrophenones produce a high percentage of extrapyramidal side effects including parkinsonism, dystonia, akathisia, and tremor. Autonomic effects are less common than with phenothiazines but include fever, tachycardia, sweating, and hypotension (rare). Cardiovascular problems, agranulocytosis, and liver impairment have been reported very rarely.

TABLE 8.7. PHENOTHIAZINES ASSOCIATED WITH HIGH INCIDENCES OF CERTAIN SIDE EFFECTS[a]

Side effects	Chlorproma-zine	Promazine	Mepazine	Fluphena-zine	Perphena-zine	Trifluopera-zine	Thioridazine
Agranulocytosis	X	X	X				
Jaundice	X	X	X				
Sedation	X						
Extrapyramidal effects				X	X	X	
Ejaculation inhibition							X
Retinal pathology							X

[a] After Klein and Davis (1969).

One unpleasant feature that the butyrophenones share with another group of drugs—the rauwolfia derivatives—is the ability to precipitate depressions; therefore their use is contraindicated in patients with a history of depression (Klerman, 1970).

Tricyclic Antidepressants

Of special note with the tricyclics are the following side effects, supplementing the material in Chapter 2.

CENTRAL NERVOUS SYSTEM

1. Fine, high-frequency tremor of the hands, arms, and head
2. Dysarthria (difficulty forming speech sounds)
3. Paresthesia (tingling sensations in arms and legs)
4. Ataxia (inability to walk)
5. Visual hallucinations (with high doses)

AUTONOMIC NERVOUS SYSTEM

1. Heart palpitations
2. Tachycardia (rapid heart beat)
3. Profuse sweating
4. Urinary retention
5. Hypotensive reaction (lowering of blood pressure)

MAO Inhibitors

LIVER TOXICITY

Early reports of serious, sometimes fatal, liver impairment led to the development of less risky types of MAO inhibitors. Liver toxicity no longer seems to be a significant problem, although patients who develop jaundice should probably be switched to another drug.

HYPERTENSIVE CRISES

It is hazardous for patients taking MAO inhibitors (Nardil, Parnate, Eutonyl, etc.) to eat foods high in tyramine content. Tyramine, a by-product of fermentation, is present in large amounts in aged cheeses, wines, and other foods where there is aging or fermentation (these are detailed in Appendix 6).

The hypertensive crisis occurs suddenly, with a severe, throbbing headache starting in the back of the head, then usually radiating forward. This is associated with elevated blood pressure, neck pain, sweating, chills, nausea, muscle twitching, and fright. When severe, there is chest pain, heart palpitations, and collapse; if associated with intracranial bleeding, this reaction may be fatal.

The incidence of hypertensive crisis is estimated to occur in approximately 3% of MAO inhibitor-treated patients. With good dietary management, however, patients should never experience these reactions.

Antianxiety Agents

Most members of this drug group produce some sedation. Often the drowsiness will dissipate spontaneously after several days of treatment. To reduce the severity of this problem, however, initial doses should be low, with a slow build-up to therapeutic levels over 4–5 days. The central nervous system depressant effects are potentiated by alcohol or barbiturates, so patients must understand that concurrent use of alcohol or other sedatives could be risky. Other CNS depressant effects may include blurred or double vision, slurred speech, lowered blood pressure, and tremor.

The risk of suicide or accidental death by the antianxiety agents is not great, except with meprobamate (Miltown, Equanil, etc.), which can be fatal in relatively small amounts. Addictive possibilities exist since these drugs do create a physiological dependence. Again, this possibility is most marked with the propanediols (meprobamate). Withdrawal symptoms are similar to barbiturate withdrawal and include anxiety, restlessness, weakness, delirium, and seizures. It should be stressed, however, that these reactions occur only when these drugs have been abused, rather than used in therapeutic dosages.

Lithium

As noted in Chapter 5, lithium can produce serious, even fatal side effects if the blood lithium levels get too high. When properly monitored, lithium side effects should be no more troublesome than side effects of any other psychotropic drug. Lithium-treated patients must keep up their dietary salt intake.

Lithium intoxication appears in several grades:

1. *Mild:* patient may be nauseated or show fine hand tremor.
2. *Moderate:* patient may exhibit gastrointestinal disturbance (anorexia, vomiting, diarrhea, upset stomach), excessive thirst, frequent urination, muscular weakness, muscle twitching, drowsiness, giddiness, coarse tremor, difficulty in walking.
3. *Advanced:* hyperactive reflexes, increased muscle tone, impaired movements, impaired consciousness, confusion, stupor, seizures, difficulty speaking, other neurological signs.
4. *Very advanced:* coma and death are possible.

Lithium should not be used in patients with kidney or cardiovascular disease, severe debilitation, or conditions requiring low-sodium diets. Concurrent use of diuretics or drugs for high blood pressure are also contraindicated. Thyroid malfunction has been observed in patients taking lithium.

The Nonmedical Practioner's Role in Monitoring Side Effects

In collaborating in the treatment of a patient taking psychotropic drugs, mental health workers should accurately report to the physician side reactions noted. Physicians are accustomed to dealing with side effects and evaluating therapeutic effect–side effect "cost–benefit ratios." Side effects are annoying and uncomfortable, sometimes serious, occasionally critical, and should never be ignored. However, in planning the drug treatment strategy for a patient, it must be remembered that unless psychotropic drugs are used in adequate dosages, they might just as well not be used at all. Homeopathic (low dosage) treatment with any psychotropic drug is unfair to the patient, unless placebo effect is specifically sought (Honigfeld, 1964a,b). It prolongs treatment unnecessarily, thereby foreclosing therapeutic planning of more appropriate drug programs. Through misguided concern for the patient's comfort, mental health workers may press for dosage reduction or discontinuation. Remember, the ineffectiveness of a low dose may make a patient feel even more hopeless. ("Not even drugs could help me.") When faced with a side effect problem, one should always consider, "In terms of psychopathology, what would this patient's condition probably be, at this time, without the drugs he is now receiving?"

If, however, the therapist has reason to think that the physician is ignoring side effects or is failing to use antiparkinson agents where they seem to be indicated, or is unwilling to talk about side effects and related problems with the patient, these concerns should be discussed openly. It is important to determine whether or not the physician has an appropriate rationale for his actions, as well as to determine whether the patient may have distorted the facts to suit his needs. In any event, a free and open discussion of such problems should be part of any collaborative therapeutic effort; if this is not forthcoming, further collaboration should be with someone else.

CHAPTER 9

DISCONTINUATION, MAINTENANCE, AND PROPHYLAXIS

In preceding chapters we have emphasized the indications for the major psychotropic drug classes in the acute and resolving stages of a variety of disorders. Important clinical questions relate also to the issue of keeping patients on long-term medication both to maintain good mental health and for possible prophylactic value in preventing recurrences of psychiatric disorder. Prolonged use of psychoactive drugs is undesirable in many ways. It is expensive and may result in numerous complications, including cardiovascular problems, liver disease, tardive dyskinesia, and retinal changes. It is also possible that prolonged use of psychiatric drugs may account for a number of unexplained deaths (Hollister and Kosek, 1965; Leetsma and Koenig, 1968). On the other hand, drug discontinuation may increase the risk of relapse. Do the benefits of long-term maintenance medication outweigh its risks? The answer to this question varies according to diagnostic group.

Schizophrenia

Although studies of drug discontinuation in schizophrenia are not numerous, the field does have the benefit of about a half dozen, well-controlled investigations. A conservative consensus from these studies is that significant clinical regression occurs in at least 40% of chronic patients removed from antipsychotic medication; in some studies, the relapse rates were in excess of 70%. Efforts at predicting the relapse-prone schizophrenic patient have been largely unsuccessful. A complete review of this field can be found in Prien and Klett (1972).

In addition to investigating the discontinuation of medication, there have been several studies of reduced or intermittent chemotherapy where various patterns of drug-free periods have been explored. Prien *et al.* (1971) reported that many long-term schizophrenic patients could get along quite well on reduced phenothiazine levels, while complete medication withdrawal resulted in severe deterioration. Under most intermittent drug patterns, relapse rate is relatively low, with the added benefit of potentially decreased side effects. In a model double-blind study of this type (Caffey *et al.*, 1964), 348 chronic schizophrenic men were studied under four conditions:

1. Continued chlorpromazine or thioridazine at maintenance levels
2. Intermittent chlorpromazine or thioridazine Monday, Wednesday, and Friday
3. Placebo daily
4. Placebo Monday, Wednesday, and Friday

After 16 weeks, 45% of the placebo patients had relapsed, 15% of the intermittent drug patients had relapsed, but only 5% of the continuously drug-treated patients relapsed.

It had been feared by some that relapsed patients would be particularly refractory to resumption of psychotropic medication. This does not seem to be the case; in general, relapsed patients exhibit symptom reduction soon after the resumption of medication.

Most drug discontinuation studies in schizophrenia have been done in chronic patients with long treatment and hospitalization histories. The need for continued phenothiazine treatment as a prophylactic measure has not been established for more acute patients or for those with histories of recurrent episodes.

Concerning maintenance phenothiazine treatment, some psychiatrists use "depot" injections of fluphenazine enanthate or fluphenazine decanoate. This is a slow-release treatment, used only once or twice a month. This form of treatment is well suited to patients who have difficulty adhering to an oral drug program, frequently a problem in case management (Rifkin et al., 1971).

Manic-Depressive Illness

The role of lithium as a prophylactic agent in cyclic manic-depressive illness is not yet fully established (Schou et al., 1970). Several studies comparing the severity and frequency of relapse before and during lithium therapy suggest that in both manic-depressive patients and recurrent depressives (without history of manic attacks) lithium is an effective prophylactic agent. Schou reported high relapse rates in depressed patients randomly assigned to placebo, compared with no relapses in lithium patients during the maintenance stage of treatment. Longitudinal studies aimed at a comparison of lithium to other psychoactive drugs are required before the relative prophylactic merits of these can be established.

To avoid risking lithium intoxication, maintenance blood levels should be kept below 1.5 mEq/liter. Scandinavian investigators suggest maintaining serum lithium levels at between .8 and 1.2 mEq/liter when lithium is used prophylactically. At these levels, typical maintenance dosages are in the range 500–1500 mg lithium carbonate daily. After a patient's condition has been stabilized by lithium, he should see his physician at least once a month for several months, Also every 2 months thereafter blood lithium levels should be obtained at each visit. Lithium is compatible with antidepressants so that the physician can consider combined therapy should the patient begin to exhibit signs of depressive relapse.

The chronic disease model is most appropriate for describing to patients the prophylactic use of lithium. It may be helpful to use the example of insulin treatment in diabetes, a chronic disease with which most people are familiar. That is, with proper medication and diet, diabetic patients remain symptom-free. Without treatment, relapse is inevitable. While the analogy to recurrent affective disorder is not perfect, it is useful in getting patients to understand (a) that the drug does not cure his recurrent illness, but rather prevents the reappearance of symptoms, and (b) if the patient fails to take his medication, relapse will likely result.

It is suggested that when the required precautions are observed, lithium can be administered indefinitely. The drug seems to have no significant effect on mental functions, and there is no evidence of withdrawal symptoms after discontinuation. After years of use, there have been no reports of habituation or altered tolerance for lithium. Although impaired thyroid function (goiter) is possible with prolonged use, this effect can probably be controlled by adjunctive medication.

Examination of the psychotropic drug literature reveals little evidence for the prophylactic action of other drugs in recurrent affective disorders.

Antidepressants

Although evidence for the efficacy of the antidepressants is clear for acute treatment, there is no solid evidence that antidepressants are effective prophylactic agents. Some psychiatrists, however, do prescribe these drugs in this manner. After successful drug treatment of the acute depressive episode with typical dosage ranges in the area 150–225 mg daily of imipramine (Tofranil), the physician then gradually tapers off the dosage. For most patients, the maintenance dosage will be in the area of half the previous therapeutic dose, continued for 6 months to 1 year.

Because of the recurrent nature of many depressions, attempts at prophylaxis with antidepressants seem reasonable. Nevertheless, good studies in support of this practice are lacking.

In the case of antidepressant treatment of panic anxiety states, there again is a lack of adequate studies, but a conservative approach would involve continued use of the effective agent at maintenance levels for 6 months to 1 year. This should ensure a relatively asymptomatic period, with the possibility of reinstituting active treatment should that be necessary.

Overview

Drug discontinuation and maintenance medication are among the least clear areas in psychopharmacology. Good evidence does exist for the prophylactic indications of the phenothiazines in chronic schizophrenia and lithium in manic-depressive illness. Chronic schizophrenic and recurrent manic-depressive patients should probably be expected to remain on a drug regimen indefinitely. This in itself represents a significant step toward the preventive treatment of two major sources of profound psychological distress. Nevertheless, evidence relating to the prophylactic indications of other drug classes in other types of patients is still unclear.

Where continued treatment is necessary and alternative treatments possible, the physician should carefully review the patient's drug history, particularly from the point of view of subjective side effects. Maintenance medication requires the patient's continued cooperation. Therefore, if possible, it is desirable to avoid using drugs which the patient rejected in the past in favor of alternate treatments which might be more acceptable.

CHAPTER 10

DRUG TREATMENT OF DRUG ADDICTION AND ALCOHOLISM

Drug therapy is a relatively new factor in the treatment of drug and alcohol abuse, and the methods to be described have not yet been adequately studied. Therefore, the reader is cautioned against unwarranted optimism, particularly since clinical experience suggests that drug and alcohol abusers are among the most difficult patients in whom to effect therapeutic change. Drug and alcohol abusers seem to develop such a generalized hunger for the substances they seek that, in addition to drug or alcohol withdrawal, long-term supportive measures are necessary to help the patient resist returning to his former habit. Therefore, rehabilitative efforts in drug and alcohol abuse must incorporate a comprehensive approach to treatment involving all appropriate therapeutic modalities. Because of the global impact drug and alcohol abuse can have on a patient's life, a comprehensive treatment program could involve participation in individual and group psychotherapy, family counseling, and vocational rehabilitation, as well as participation in lay group activities such as Alcoholics Anonymous or one of the many self-help programs for drug abusers.

It is beyond the scope of this book to consider all these approaches to the treatment of drug and alcohol abuse. Rather, we will be concerned here only with those aspects of treatment involving drug therapy. For most patients this should represent only a small part of a total treatment program.

Heroin Dependency

Formerly, the typical heroin addict was a ghetto resident; now, he is seen increasingly in all social strata. Heroin addicts usually develop both a psychological as well as a physical dependency on the drug, along with a tolerance to its effects, such that increasing doses are necessary to produce the desired physical and psychological effects. The heroin (or other opiate) abuser's total preoccupation with drug taking eventually results in personal neglect, poor nourishment, and a high risk of infection from injections with contaminated materials. The high cost of supporting an illicit drug habit almost inevitably leads to a life of crime which is hazardous both to the abuser and to society. If heroin substitutes (such as methadone) did nothing else but replace an underworld supplier with a low-cost, government source of drugs, a significant step will have been taken toward the reduction of crime. In actual practice, the situation is somewhat more complex. Since methadone taken orally does not produce the same euphoriant qualities as heroin, some addicts will use it only as a last resort to prevent withdrawal symptoms. If money is available, they prefer to buy heroin. However, some addicts have found that oral methadone "shot up" produces a euphoriant effect similar to that of heroin. This newly discovered property has enhanced methadone's popularity among addicts. Consequently, some methadone is being sold illicitly.

The management problems of opiate abuse can be considered at three levels: (*a*) toxic overdose, (*b*) withdrawal syndromes and (*c*) rehabilitation of the chronic heroin addict.

The problem of treating toxic overdoses is beyond the province of psychiatric care and is typically dealt with by the internist or neurologist. The nonmedical practitioner should simply be aware of the life-threatening nature of such overdose conditions (see Chapter 12 for a more complete discussion of drug emergencies).

Opiate withdrawal is an uncomfortable but not life-threatening syndrome which may begin within a few hours after the last dose and may continue for 1 or 2 days. Treatment of the withdrawal syndrome is best accomplished in a hospital setting but can frequently be handled on an outpatient basis; with the heroin substitute methadone the patient can be gradually weaned from the drug, rather than forced to stop "cold turkey."

In treating heroin withdrawal, the physician will typically withhold treatment to watch for the onset of withdrawal symptoms. These may include runny nose; sweating; nausea; diarrhea; increases in blood pressure, body temperature, and respiration rate; anxiety; generalized body aches; and restlessness. If such symptoms do not begin to appear within 36 hours for heroin addicts or 48–72 hours for persons on methadone maintenance, the withdrawal syndrome is not expected to develop at all, and the patient is not considered physiologically addicted. With the appearance of withdrawal symptoms, methadone therapy is begun until the symptoms are stabilized and methadone decreased gradually each day over a period of up to 1 week, until a permanent, maintenance dosage level is achieved.

Once the patient is successfully withdrawn from drugs, he will experience no further withdrawal symptoms; yet, if released back to the street without continued treatment, he can be expected within a short time to again seek to satisfy his opiate hunger, raising money through crime or prostitution in many cases.

At present, there are two main approaches to the long-term drug therapy of the opiate abuser. Both of these require high motivation on the part of addicts in order to remain in treatment.

Since the problem of keeping a former drug abuser off drugs is so great, the possibility of alternative forms of chemical therapy have an inherent appeal. Currently, the major chemical approaches to the treatment of drug abuse are of two types: (*a*) the use of heroin substitutes, and (*b*) the use of heroin antagonists.

The best-developed program of heroin substitution is the methadone maintenance program developed by Dole and Nyswander (1966). This program begins with the hospitalized patient being treated with methadone. The dosage is increased once or twice a week in periodic increments over a 4–6 week period until the patient is receiving a single, oral dose of 80–120 mg per day (usually administered in fruit juice). Concurrent activites include urine screening for detection of illicit drug use, as well as vocational and educational rehabilitation. Because many heroin abusers are quite willing to trade methadone for heroin, addicts should not be trusted to self-administer methadone. They should be required to come to a clinic where the drug can be individually administered in liquid form, under observation. This form of treatment has the advantage of being simple and reportedly successful in a substantial proportion of cases so treated.

The disadvantages of methadone maintenance are principally that methadone is a narcotic and, therefore, addicting. Furthermore, some addicts may object to having to remain "drugged." Dole and Nyswander presume that hard core heroin addicts have to be maintained for life on methadone, and in that sense the patient can hardly be considered "cured," but rather "controlled" or "stabilized." Also controversial in the Dole and Nyswander method is the high methadone dosage levels that they use. They feel that about 100 mg per day of methadone not only eliminates the hunger for heroin, but also serves to block the effects of heroin if it is used.

Cyclazocine and naloxone are heroin antagonists which block the effects of heroin. The most dramatic example of this is that administration of cyclazocine to an addict on heroin will immediately precipitate a full-blown withdrawal syndrome. Furthermore, a former addict taking cyclazocine will not get any effect from heroin. Typically, treatment with cyclazocine involves withdrawal from narcotics and an initial treatment with cyclazocine at 0.25 mg daily, increased by 0.25 mg every other day until an effective dosage of about 4 mg per day is reached.

The principal advantage of cyclazocine and naloxone is that they are not narcotics, and many addicts may find this preferable to being "drugged" on methadone. A major disadvantage of these treatments is that they do not block the heroin hunger. In addition, there may be significant side effects during the initial administration, including perceptual distortion, restlessness, and increased sex drive. Nevertheless, these symptoms can usually be managed with a temporary dosage reduction. A further disadvantage is the relatively short duration of action (approximately 18 hours for cyclazocine and 3 hours for naloxone); however, long-acting forms are under development.

All the opiate substitutes and antagonists are cumbersome treatment methods, requiring frequent clinic visits and very highly motivated patients to adhere successfully to such therapeutic programs. For the majority of addicts, these methods are impractical.

Amphetamine Abuse

Amphetamines, or "ups," are widely used because of their transient, euphoriant effects, as well as the feeling of mental alertness produced by their occasional use. Thus, while many individuals develop a psychological dependency on these drugs, with increased use the desirable effects tend to disappear, giving way to various symptoms including jitteriness, irritability, difficulty in concentration, loss of appetite, and loss of libido. Some users, particularly those taking these drugs intravenously, develop full-blown paranoid psychoses which persist well beyond the time the drugs themselves would be expected to remain active in the body.

It has been found that the phenothiazines are antagonists of amphetamines, as well as of other hallucinogenic agents such as LSD. Therefore, patients experiencing amphetamine reactions should be treated with a phenothiazine. It has also been suggested that patients with a propensity for periodic amphetamine abuse be premedicated with a phenothiazine as a means of blocking any effect which subsequent amphetamine use might have.

In reviewing the treatment of such patients, one should always bear in mind that many amphetamine abusers are really "garbage-heads," that is, individuals who will indiscriminately ingest a wide variety of chemical substances. It would obviously be a mistake, then, to concentrate on one feature of the patient's drug abuse problem (such as amphetamine abuse) if there is a history of multiple drug abuse.

Barbiturate Dependency

Chronic barbiturate users develop both a psychological and physical dependency on continued drug use. Tolerance to barbiturates develops so that there is a tendency for barbiturate users gradually to increase drug intake. Accidental death among barbiturate users is not uncommon. It can occur even more readily when these drugs are used in combination with alcohol.

Withdrawal symptoms include feelings of anxiety, muscle twitching, tremor, muscular weakness, dizziness, disturbed vision, nausea and vomiting, insomnia, and decreased blood pressure. Seizure, delirium, coma, and death are possible. Withdrawal symptoms begin approximately 24 hours after the last dose and effects are maximal 2–3 days later, slowly subsiding thereafter.

The treatment of choice is gradual weaning, using one of the barbiturates, preferably pentobarbital. Because there are serious risks associated with barbiturate withdrawal, this process should take place in a hospital setting where close observation is possible and where the weaning schedule can be very gradual. If withdrawal symptoms reappear during this period, they should be handled by a slight, temporary increase in barbiturate dosage.

The utility of drug treatment for the barbiturate user is indeed extremely limited. Appropriate use of barbiturates during the withdrawal period can greatly ease the patient's discomfort as well as decrease his serious medical risk. Nevertheless, long-term rehabilitation remains a difficult task, potentially involving the skills of a variety of mental health workers.

Alcohol Abuse

In many ways alcohol abuse resembles barbiturate abuse, with the development of psychological and physical dependency, as well as tolerance to the substance. The timing of the withdrawal syndrome is similar to that of barbiturates—beginning about 24 hours after the last drink, peaking within 2–3 days, with subsequent, slow improvement. Withdrawal symptoms include most notably tremulousness, seizures, delirium, and perceptual distortion. Studies suggest that antianxiety agents such as chlordiazepoxide may be of some help in the management of alcohol withdrawal states.

As an added feature, chronic alcohol use carries with it the risk of tissue damage, particularly to the central nervous system and liver. Nutritional disturbances are a frequent accompaniment to chronic alcoholism, with the carbohydrates provided by alcohol taking the place of a regular diet.

Concerning the long-term treatment of the chronic alcoholic, the major chemical treatment alternatives are either Antabuse (disulfiram) or for those patients who use alcohol as a means of reducing anxiety, one of the benzodiazepine antianxiety agents. Chemical treatment of alcoholism has been notably unsuccessful, however.

Antabuse premedication produces a horrible reaction in the patient who drinks any alcohol. Typically, the patient becomes flushed, experiences very rapid heartbeat, a feeling of fearfulness, pounding headache, and rapid breathing. Within a few minutes his blood pressure drops and he becomes weak, dizzy, and nauseated, with vomiting and fainting occurring. This reaction may last for several hours.

The Antabuse treatment is typically begun in the hospital starting at 500 mg a day for 4 or 5 days, with the dose dropping to 250 mg daily thereafter. Some clinicians believe it useful to have an alcohol trial prior to the patient's leaving the hospital. He is warned about the effects of mixing alcohol and Antabuse and is instructed to drink half an ounce of alcohol. The effects are immediate, dramatic, and unpleasant, and the patient may feel ill for several hours. Other clinicians feel that a serious warning is sufficient in itself. Obviously, a treatment as noxious as Antabuse can be effective only for those patients who seriously attempt to end their drinking problem.

Patients on Antabuse must be warned against the dangers of alcohol in any form including medicines, as an ingredient in cooked food, and in industrial fumes. This is not an innocuous procedure, and the patient placed on Antabuse must be carefully evaluated medically prior to treatment.

Overview

Review of the field of drug treatment in drug and alcohol abuse leads one to conclude that there are at present several significant chemical aids in the treatment of these disorders. Nevertheless, no one of these in itself represents a total treatment program for any type of addiction problem. The area of greatest promise and probably the area of greatest research activity is in the treatment of opiate addiction. Heroin substitutes and antagonists which take the "kick" out of drug use are effective in eliminating heroin use, but only in motivated patients. Such treatments, however, are annoying and require frequent clinic visits. With the anticipated development of improved heroin antagonists, a long-acting naloxone, for example, a larger proportion of heroin addicts may become treatable.

Chronic barbiturate and amphetamine abuse seem to be problems without the promise of rapid resolution. However, additional steps to curb the current, widespread distribution of these compounds might be useful in protecting the young.

Alcohol abuse is perhaps the most extensive of all the disorders we have considered. Because of the wide acceptance and accessibility of alcohol, it is not possible to turn off the source of supply. With alcohol use such an established part of our culture, nonabusers would certainly not tolerate any attempts at inhibiting its distribution. For the alcoholic, drug treatment, aside from Antabuse, holds little promise of help. However, this treatment is so noxious that only the most highly motivated patient could be expected to endure it.

CHAPTER 11

CURRENT DEVELOPMENTS

A number of new developments in clinical psychopharmacology are worthy of mention. Because these developments are new and the supporting research is neither complete nor adequate, these topics have been gathered here so that the ideas they represent can be clearly identified as tentative.

NEW ANTIPSYCHOTIC DRUG CLASSES

Under active clinical testing are several members of two new antipsychotic drug classes, the dibenzodiazepines and diphenylbutylalanines. This latter group includes pimozide, fluspirilene and penfluridal. The dibenzodiazepines include clothiapine, clozapine, loxapine and metiapine, all of which appear to be effective antipsychotic agents. Each of these is being tested clinically, with encouraging early reports.

TRICYCLIC – THYROID SYNERGISM

It has been suggested by Prange *et al.* (1970) that the rather slow therapeutic response time of the tricyclic antidepressants (2–3 weeks for partial effect and 3–6 weeks for full effect) might be accelerated with concurrent use of thyroid medication. Substantiation of this finding could represent a significant modification in the customary manner of prescribing antidepressants, with very beneficial effects for patients. However, there have not yet been good, independent cross-validation studies. Clinical impressions by others of a small number of cases have been only partially supportive, suggesting that this effect may be unique to females.

ANTIDEPRESSANTS IN HYSTEROID–DYSPHORIC STATES

Klein (1972) has described a class of patients characterized as "hysteroid–dysphoric." Principally adolescent or young adult female patients, they are usually considered hysterics or neurotic depressives by other investigators. Klein has singled them out as a diagnostic entity because as a group they exhibit marked, positive responses to MAO inhibitor antidepressants. The reactive aspect of these patients' mood fluctuations is particularly significant, especially in relation to the quality of their heterosexual interactions. Their strong need for demonstrations of affection from boyfriend or spouse is matched by an equally strong rejection sensitivity. Marked mood fluctuations occur in response to daily variations in perceived affection or rejection by heterosexual partners.

On phenelzine (Nardil), such patients frequently exhibit marked stabilization of mood, particularly reduction in the depressive reactions resulting from actual or perceived interpersonal rejection. After mood is stabilized, hysteroid-dysphoric patients may require long-term treatment with an MAO inhibitor, at reduced dosage. When effective, this treatment can produce rather dramatic changes in the patient's often previously erratic and unstable life style. While there is little supporting research concerning the use of MAO inhibitors in this patient group, the possibilities are intriguing. An illustrative case may be found in Klein and Howard (1972).

USE OF ANTICONVULSANTS IN PATIENTS WITH IMPULSE DISORDERS

Several converging lines of evidence from different investigators point to the probability that for many patients with problems of impulse control there is likely a component of abnormal brain function. Most often implicated is the limbic system, a diffuse neural network located deep within the temporal lobes (amygdaloid-hippocampal complex). Activity in these areas is associated with a variety of emotional experiences. Experimental stimulation within the limbic system produces rage and attack behavior, usually with well-coordinated muscular activity. It is hypothesized that in man, subcortical seizures (uncontrolled bursts of electrical activity) in limbic system areas may produce altered states of awareness in which impulse control is significantly impaired. These states resemble psychomotor epileptic attacks except that the aggressive, sometimes homicidal acts are carried out more skillfully. In addition, there is sometimes an extended prodromal period before the actual "seizure," when the patient may become preoccupied with aggressive fantasies which in some cases seem to function as rehearsals for the ultimate aggressive performance itself. Mark and Ervin's book *Violence and the Brain* (1970) is a particularly stimulating introduction to this field.

Monroe (1969) has attempted to integrate these findings, summarizing experiences with neurosurgical as well as with chemical intervention methods. While neurosurgical approaches are beyond the scope of this book and are themselves in a very early stage of development, there is some research supporting the utility of anticonvulsant agents (e.g., Dilantin or Mysoline) in treating such patients.

Because of these promising findings, interest in this field is growing. Much current work is aimed at developing more refined diagnostic methods. Particularly significant is the effort to refine brain wave (EEG or electroencephalographic) recording. As advances in this field are made, further research will likely aim at relating specific anticonvulsant drugs to specific types of brain abnormality. At present, this work is proceeding, with some success, entirely on a clinical level.

Relationships between brain development and impulse control are especially marked in children, adolescents, and young adults. With increasing age, young patients may show both a regularization of brain wave abnormalities and decreased "acting out" behavior. It is possible that certain hard-to-treat teenagers with poor impulse control could be helped through anticonvulsant drug treatment. With this group of patients, a sophisticated and adventurous neurologist, epileptologist, or neuropsychiatrist could prove to be a useful collaborator.

HYPERACTIVE CHILDREN

Hyperactive children can very often be helped by a regimen of stimulant drugs, which are frequently effective in making them amenable to instruction at school. Because the stimulant drugs exhibit a paradoxical calming effect in the preadolescent period, there is little danger of "hooking" children on these drugs. It should be understood that stimulants are indicated for hyperactivity only in children between the ages 6–12, whose hyperactivity make the school experience intolerable for the child, his schoolmates, and his teachers.

There is some evidence that hyperactive children with learning disorders can also be helped with phenothiazines. Controlled studies in this area are now underway and appear promising.

SCHOOL PHOBIA

Extension of earlier work demonstrating the efficacy of antidepressant agents in panic states in adults led to the exploration of using these drugs in children whose extreme fear of attending school severely restricts their social and educational development. Current, controlled investigations have encouraging preliminary results (Gittelman-Klein and Klein, 1971). Although there has been great concern expressed in the lay press over the inhumanities of "drugging" children, if the present results are ultimately confirmed such criticisms would be clearly unfounded since many children seem to improve so vastly when treated psychopharmacologically. This use of drugs in children must be evaluated in the context of each child's intellectual, physical, and social problems.

AFFECTIVE DISORDER IN CHILDREN AND ADOLESCENTS

Studies by Annell (1969) and Frommer (1968) suggest that lithium may be useful in treating children with affective *equivalents* of adult hypomania. Such children exhibit aimless, restless activity, disconnected conversation, and grossly impaired ability to concentrate. Lithium seems to help some of these children, as well as others with somatic complaints and severe temper outbursts.

As noted in Chapter 3, phenothiazines effectively modulate the marked mood swings of emotionally unstable adolescents. Lithium also appears promising in this area (Rifkin *et al.*, 1972).

GERIATRIC PSYCHOPHARMACOLOGY

There has been limited but growing interest in the identification of certain drugs within each major class which may be particularly benign with regard to those side effects that are most troublesome to geriatric patients. This is especially important in populations at high risk for cardiovascular difficulties. In one study of geriatric schizophrenics, acetophenazine (Tindal) produced fewer side effects than trifluoperazine (Stelazine) (Honigfeld *et al.*, 1965).

Potentially marked hypotensive effects of antidepressant agents make the geriatric group particularly vulnerable to these drugs. Because of the growing numbers of geriatric patients being treated in both institutional and outpatient settings, further developments along these lines are likely.

Tic Douloureux (Trigeminal Neuralgia)

Carbamazepine (Tegretol), a drug structurally similar to imipramine (Tofranil), seems to be useful in the treatment of *tic douloureux*, a condition in which there is severe, intractable facial pain, usually in the area of the cheek.

Gilles de la Tourette's Syndrome

Gilles de la Tourette's syndrome is characterized by body and facial tics, barking sounds, and compulsive cursing (coprolalia), usually starting in childhood. Frequently diagnosed as functional or hysterical, it is probably a neurological disorder. Haloperidol appears to be a specific treatment affording a high degree of symptomatic improvement. In a recent review, over 80% of haloperidol-treated cases were helped, compared with less than 40% for all other forms of treatment (Snyder *et al.*, 1970).

New Drug Developments

Drug companies are always exploring new drug classes as well as molecular variations within existing drug classes, in order to produce more effective drugs with reduced side effects. The Psychopharmacology Research Branch of the National Institute of Mental Health has a very active program of early clinical drug evaluations aimed at objectively evaluating some of the new compounds developed by the drug houses. This program supports the work of highly qualified investigators, all of whom use a common set of evaluative instruments, including the BPRS psychiatric rating scale

(Overall and Gorham, 1962) and the NOSIE-30 ward behavior scale (Honigfeld *et al.*, 1966); this ensures comparability of findings between investigators. While the majority of such evaluations end in scientific *cul-de-sacs*, nevertheless, some promising new compounds do emerge.

There is growing interest in new long-acting forms of existing drugs. Because many out-patients cannot be counted on to take their prescribed medication regularly, the introduction of long-acting injectable and oral preparations has been very well received. Furthermore, the added costs incurred by frequent dosing provide an added incentive for the development of long-acting drugs. At present, there are two major types of delayed dosage forms. Sustained release capsules or tablets consist of drug pellets with varying disintegration rates—these are said to distribute dosage over the course of a day, eliminating the need for divided doses. However, since most psychiatric drugs can be given as a single daily dose, these formulations are not too useful. "Depot" injections (such as fluphenazine enanthate) which can be given as infrequently as once every 2 to 4 weeks are very popular, particularly in the management of patients on long-term maintenance treatment.

MEGAVITAMIN THERAPY

Backed by a strenuous public relations effort, Drs. Humphrey Osmond and Abraham Hoffer have been heralding the virtues of vitamin therapy in schizophrenia. Except for the relatively small number of patients suffering from organic psychoses associated with marked physical debilitation, metabolic, or nutritional defect (e.g., pellagra), there is as yet no good confirming evidence that vitamins are an efficacious treatment form for psychosis in general.

CHAPTER 12

HANDLING DRUG EMERGENCIES

Because drug emergencies are medical problems, ultimate responsibility for handling these situations lies in medical hands. Playing physician is a serious professional indiscretion, and one that could prove costly should a disgruntled patient or family member press for court action. However, an important aspect of responsible professional practice is knowing how to recognize and handle drug emergencies—knowing when to refer a problem back to the physician's attention versus calling directly for emergency assistance.

There are two major types of potential drug emergencies: (*a*) side effects and (*b*) overdose.

Serious Side Effects

In a collaborative relationship with a physician, the nonmedical practitioner may have more face-to-face patient contact, and should, therefore, be attuned to patients' reports of possible side effects. Side effects should be called to the treating physician's attention and reevaluated in future contacts with the patient. As reviewed in Chapter 8, most side reactions, while troublesome, are not seriously life-threatening.

Potentially serious or life-threatening reactions require vigorous action. Bear in mind that while side effects *in general* are dose-related, this is not always true. Therefore, one can never ignore side effects as insignificant, merely because a patient is on a low dose.

Of the serious side effects, several bear special mention:

1. Agranulocytosis
2. Liver involvement
3. Lithium toxicity
4. Hypertensive crises
5. Dystonic reactions

Agranulocytosis is rare but serious. Patients taking phenothiazines who report sore throat and sudden, unexplained, severe fatigue, particularly if associated with fever, should be referred immediately for a medical examination which should include blood testing. These symptoms could turn out to be nothing more than a passing infection but, on the other hand, they might be symptoms of agranulocytosis.

Liver involvement is also associated with feelings of fatigue and general malaise, especially appetite loss. Most suggestive, of course, is yellow, jaundiced skin and eyes. This, too, requires immediate referral back to the physician, who will almost certainly discontinue medication if liver toxicity is suspected.

Lithium toxicity is graded on several levels of severity, as detailed in Chapter 5. Attention to all signs of unwanted central nervous system effects is always warranted, but is especially important for patients on lithium. Because of the toxic hazards of lithium, signs of central nervous system difficulty (see Chapter 8) should not be minimized, but reported promptly to the treating physician.

Hypertensive crises can occur in association with the taking of any MAO inhibitor antidepressant. As described in Chapter 8, eating foods high in tyramine content (see Appendix 6) can precipitate hypertensive or hypotensive crises. The typical MAO inhibitor-induced hypertensive headache should be referred promptly to the physician. Hypertensive crises are immediately life-threatening, and the patient's welfare demands emergency attention. If a patient taking an MAO inhibitor is found unconscious or in a stuporous or comatose condition, he must immediately be taken to a hospital. Call the hospital or the police first; next call the treating physician; then call responsible family members if they are not aware of the problem.

When making the emergency call, *stress* to the hospital or police authorities that the patient is taking an MAO inhibitor and therefore certain *pressor agents such as adrenalin (epinephrine) must not be used* in treating the patient. (Norepinephrine is an acceptable alternative.) Pressor agents may react with MAO inhibitors to induce or increase intracranial bleeding, which at least would be harmful, and could prove fatal.

Dystonic reactions are not usually severe, but when the head and neck muscles become rigid and contorted, with breathing or swallowing difficulties, there may not be time to call the physician before calling for an ambulance. Such patients require intramuscular antiparkinson agents, such as Kemadrin (procyclidine), Cogentin (benztropine), Artane (trihexyphenidyl) or Akineton (biperiden). If the dystonia is severe, intravenous antihistamines can be used, perhaps more safely than the antiparkinson agents. If the patient's physician can be contacted quickly, he may be able to pass this information along to the hospital emergency room personnel. If not, it is the non-medical practitioner's responsibility to indicate what the problem might be, suggesting that intramuscular antiparkinson drugs or intravenous antihistamines be used.

Overdose

Drug overdoses, whether intentional or accidental, should always be regarded seriously. Typically, a therapist will learn of an overdose by a phone call from the patient. Handling this telephone call is critical because once the connection is broken, it may be impossible to get additional, needed information. Therefore, as soon as you realize that there is a possible overdose patient on the phone do the following:

1. Ask for the *phone number* patient is calling from (this can help to determine patient's location, if necessary)
2. Ask for patient's *exact location* (including apartment or room number, name on mail box or doorbell, etc.)
3. Determine *type of drugs* taken and *quantity*, if possible
4. Instruct patient to force himself to *vomit* by sticking fingers, pencil, spoon, etc., into back of throat (try to get him to vomit into a pot, bowl, or other container which can go with him to the hospital for examination)
5. *Call police* or emergency number (preferably on another line, while holding open line to patient) and send help out immediately
6. Try to keep the patient *on the line* and indicate that you are trying to help him
7. If patient is still on line and does not know name of drugs taken, try to get a *description*, and look this up in Appendix 4 (tablets) or Appendix 5 (capsules)
8. Follow up with police or hospital, passing along information on possible drugs taken, so that proper emergency treatment can be performed [if MAO inhibitors are involved, instruct that *pressor agents are contraindicated* (norepinephrine is acceptable)]
9. Contact family members or other responsible parties if possible

Under no circumstances should an overdose victim be told to drive himself anywhere. This is a serious hazard to the patient and to others. Tell the patient to stay where he is, that help is on the way. Do not be reluctant about calling the police or hospital. Failure to seek such help for the patient at such times is professionally irresponsible. Furthermore, proper handling of a drug emergency can enhance the status of the mental health worker in the patient's eyes, thereby facilitating therapeutic work after the medical emergency has passed.

CHAPTER **13**

DIAGNOSIS AND SOMATIC TREATMENT

The purpose of this chapter is to provide an overview of the indications and contraindications for somatic treatment across the full spectrum of psychiatric disorders. This will be done by reference to a set of tables organized according to the latest American Psychiatric Association Diagnostic and Statistical Manual (DSM-II), the "official" United States psychiatric nomenclature.

The tables are set up in code number order showing every possible diagnosis cross-tabulated against the major drug classes (plus ECT). The symbols in the body of Tables 13.1–13.5 stand for *definitely indicated* (+ + +), *indicated* (+ +), *possibly indicated* (+), and *contraindicated* (−). Contraindications are noted only where the use of a particular treatment form might be expected to result in deterioration in the patient's condition. Most of the cells in Tables 13.1–13.5 are blank, meaning that somatic treatments are neither indicated nor contraindicated.

Summary tables of this sort are necessarily limited, substituting breadth of coverage for depth. The reader should refer to the appropriate earlier chapters for more complete discussions of indications and contraindications for the major classes of somatic treatment.

TABLE 13.1. Psychotropic Drug Indications and Contraindications for Organic Brain Syndromes (APA Diagnoses 290.0–294.8)

Code	Diagnosis	Antipsychotics	Antidepressants	Anti-anxiety	Lithium	Stimulants	Sedatives	Anticonvulsants	ECT	Other
	Senile and presenile dementia									
290.0	Senile dementia	+ +								
290.1	Presenile dementia	+ +								
	Alcoholic psychosis									
291.0	Delirium tremens			+ + +				+ + + (if convulsing)		
291.1	Korsakov's psychosis									
291.2	Other alcoholic hallucinations	+								
291.3	Alcohol paranoid state	+								
291.4	Acute alcohol intoxication									
291.5	Alcoholic deterioration									
291.6	Pathological intoxication									
291.9	Other alcoholic psychosis									
	Psychosis associated with intracranial infection									
292.0	General paralysis	+								
292.1	Syphilis of central nervous system	+								
292.2	Epidemic encephalitis									

Code	Condition					
292.3	Other and unspecified encephalitis	+				
292.9	Other intracranial infection	+				
	Psychosis associated with other cerebral condition					
293.0	Cerebral arteriosclerosis	+			–	
293.1	Other cerebrovascular disturbance	+			–	
293.2	Epilepsy	+	+			++
293.3	Intracranial neoplasm					+++
293.4	Degenerative disease of the CNS					
293.5	Brain trauma					
293.9	Other cerebral condition					
	Psychosis associated with other physical condition					
294.0	Endocrine disorder					
294.1	Metabolic and nutritional disorder					
294.2	Systemic infection					
294.3	Drug or poison intoxication (other than alcohol)	++				
294.4	Childbirth	++	+			+
294.8	Other and unspecified physical condition	+				

TABLE 13.2. Psychotropic Drug Indications and Contraindications for Psychosis Not Attributable to Physical Condition

(APA Diagnoses 295.0–298.0)

Code	Diagnosis	Antipsychotics	Antidepressants	Antianxiety	Lithium	Stimulants	Sedatives	Anticonvulsants	ECT	Other
	Schizophrenia									
295.0	Simple	+++	−			−				
295.1	Hebephrenic	+++	−			−				
295.2	Catatonic	+++	−			−				
295.23	Catatonic type, excited	+++							++	
295.24	Catatonic type, withdrawn	+++							++	
295.3	Paranoid	+++	−			−				
295.4	Acute schizophrenic episode	+++	−			−				
295.5	Latent	+++	−			−				
295.6	Residual	+++	−			−				
295.7	Schizo-affective	+++	−		+	−				
295.73	Schizo-affective, excited	+++			+	−			++	
295.74	Schizo-affective depressed	+++	+			−			++	
295.8	Childhood	++	−			−				
295.90	Chronic undifferentiated	++	−			−				

295.99	Other schizophrenia					
	Major affective disorders					
296.0	Involutional melancholia	++	++		+	++
296.1	Manic-depressive illness, manic	+++		+++	−	
296.2	Manic-depressive illness, depressed	+	++	+		++
296.3	Manic-depressive illness, circular	++	+	+++	−	
296.33	Manic-depressive, circular, manic	+++		+++	−	
296.34	Manic-depressive, circular, depressed	++	++	+		
296.8	Other major affective disorder					++
	Paranoid states					
297.0	Paranoia	++				
297.1	Involutional paranoid states	++				
297.9	Other paranoid state	++				
	Other psychoses					
298.0	Psychotic depressive reaction	+	+++			+++

TABLE 13.3. Psychotropic Drug Indications and Contraindications for Neuroses and Personality Disorders

(APA Diagnoses 300.0–304.8)

Code	Diagnosis	Antipsychotics	Antidepressants	Anti-anxiety	Lithium	Stimulants	Sedatives	Anticonvulsants	ECT	Other
	Neuroses									
300.0	Anxiety	+		+++		−	−			
300.1	Hysterical		−			−	−			
300.13	Hysterical, conversion type	−	−			−				
300.14	Hysterical, dissociative type	−				−	−			
300.2	Phobic		+	++						
300.3	Obsessive compulsive		+							
300.4	Depressive	+	+							
300.5	Neurasthenic									
300.6	Depersonalization									
300.7	Hypochondriacal			+						
300.8	Other neurosis									
	Personality disorders									
301.0	Paranoid									
301.1	Cyclothymic	++			+	−	−			
301.2	Schizoid									

112

301.3	Explosive	+
301.4	Obsessive compulsive	
301.5	Hysterical	++
301.6	Asthenic	
301.7	Antisocial	
301.81	Passive-aggressive	
301.82	Inadequate	
301.89	Other specified types	
	Sexual deviation	
302.0	Homosexuality	
302.1	Fetishism	
302.2	Pedophilia	
302.3	Transvestism	
302.4	Exhibitionism	
302.5	Voyeurism	
302.6	Sadism	
302.7	Masochism	
302.8	Other sexual deviation	
	Alcoholism	
303.0	Episodic excessive drinking	Antabuse
303.1	Habitual excessive drinking	Antabuse
303.2	Alcohol addiction	Antabuse
303.9	Other alcoholism	Antabuse

113

TABLE 13.3—(*Continued*)

Code	Diagnosis	Antipsy-chotics	Antide-pressants	Anti-anxiety	Lithium	Stimu-lants	Sedatives	Anticon-vulsants	ECT	Other
	Drug Dependence									
304.0	Opium, opium alkaloids, and their derivatives									Metha-done, Naloxone, etc.
304.1	Synthetic analgesics with morphinelike effects									Metha-done, Naloxone, etc.
304.2	Barbiturates									
304.3	Other hypnotics and sedatives or "tranquilizers"			+						
304.4	Cocaine					−				
304.5	*Cannabis sativa* (hashish, marihuana)									
304.6	Other psychostimulants	+								
304.7	Hallucinogens	+ +								
304.8	Other drug dependence									

114

TABLE 13.4. Psychotropic Drug Indications and Contraindications for Miscellaneous Diagnoses (APA Diagnoses 305.0–309.)

Code	Diagnosis	Antipsychotics	Antidepressants	Anti-anxiety	Lithium	Stimulants	Sedatives	Anticonvulsants	ECT	Other
	Psychophysiologic disorders									
305.0	Skin			++						
305.1	Musculoskeletal			+++						
305.2	Respiratory			++						
305.3	Cardiovascular			++						
305.4	Hemic and lymphatic			++						
305.5	Gastro-intestinal			++						
305.6	Genito-urinary									
305.7	Endocrine									
305.8	Organ of special sense									
305.9	Other type									
	Special symptoms									
306.0	Speech disturbance									
306.1	Specific learning disturbance									
306.2	Tic									Carbamazepine for tic douloureux
306.3	Other psychomotor disorder									

TABLE 13.4— (*Continued*)

Code	Diagnosis	Anti-psychotics	Antide-pressants	Anti-anxiety	Lithium	Stimu-lants	Seda-tives	Anticon-vulsants	ECT	Other
306.4	Disorders of sleep			+ +			+ +			
306.5	Feeding disturbance			+ +						
306.6	Enuresis		+							
306.7	Encopresis									
306.8	Cephalalgia									
306.9	Other special symptoms									
	Transient situational disturbances									
307.0	Adjustment reaction of infancy									
307.1	Adjustment reaction of childhood									
307.2	Adjustment reaction of adolescence									
307.3	Adjustment reaction of adult life									
307.4	Adjustment reaction of late life									
	Behavior disorders childhood and adolescence									
308.0	Hyperkinetic reaction	+ +				+ + +				
308.1	Withdrawing reaction									
308.2	Overanxious reaction			+ +						
308.3	Runaway reaction									

116

308.4	Unsocialized aggressive reaction	
308.5	Group delinquent reaction	
308.9	Other reaction	
	Nonpsychotic OBS[a]	
309.0	Intracranial infection	
309.13	Alcohol (simple drunkenness)	
309.14	Other drug, poison or systemic intoxication	
309.2	Brain trauma	
309.3	Circulatory disturbance	
309.4	Epilepsy	+++
309.5	Disturbance of metabolism, growth or nutrition	
309.6	Senile or presenile brain disease	
309.7	Intracranial neoplasm	
309.8	Degenerative disease of the CNS	
309.9	Other physical condition	

[a] All these conditions may be associated with nonpsychotic agitation, for which antipsychotic drugs may be helpful; these conditions may also be associated with depression, for which antidepressants may be useful.

117

TABLE 13.5. Psychotropic Drug Indications and Contraindications for Mental Retardation (APA Diagnoses 310.–315.)

Code	Diagnosis	Antipsy-chotics	Antide-pressants	Anti anxiety	Lithium	Stimu-lants	Seda-tives	Anticon-vulsants	ECT	Other
	Mental retardation									
310.0	Borderline									
311.0	Mild									
312.0	Moderate									
313.0	Severe									
314.0	Profound									
315.0	Unspecified									
	With each: following or associated with									
.0	Infection or intoxication									
.1	Trauma or physical agent									
.2	Disorders of metabolism, growth or nutrition									
.3	Gross brain disease (postnatal)									
.4	Unknown prenatal influence									
.5	Chromosomal abnormality									
.6	Prematurity									
.7	Major psychiatric disorder									
.8	Psychosocial (environ-mental) deprivation									
.9	Other condition									

Treat appropriately for associated disorder (see Tables 13.1–13.4).

Review of these tables shows clearly that the major indications for somatic therapy are in the treatment of the "functional" psychoses. These are the serious, debilitating disorders where etiology is still poorly understood. Nevertheless, many such patients can for the first time be treated, rather than be managed custodially. In addition, the psychiatrist now has a chemical mechanism for relieving that ubiguitous source of psychological distress, anticipatory anxiety. Furthermore, one can see the beginnings of a new era of preventive psychiatry evidenced by the prophylactic use of lithium in manic-depressive patients.

CHAPTER 14

EVALUATING YOUR MEDICAL COLLEAGUES

Having completed this review of the state of the psychopharmacologic arts, the reader should now be better able to assess the quality of psychiatric drug practice. To facilitate this process, this chapter provides an evaluation of 19 aspects of psychopharmacologic practice which can usefully be considered when evaluating the work of one's medical colleagues.

LOW-DOSAGE MEDICATION

Perhaps the most common error made in the prescription of psychotropic drugs is the use of inadequate dosage levels. Many physicians seem to share with their patients the irrational belief that somatic treatment is second class treatment: nothing could be further from the truth. Withholding antidepressant medication from the seriously depressed patient is analogous to withholding insulin from the diabetic. Where indicated, psychotropic drugs are an essential, although not necessarily exclusive, part of the total treatment program.

However, the uncertain physician may express his ambivalence by prescribing drugs at inadequate dosage levels. Tables 2.1, 3.1, and 4.1 provide rough guidelines to adult therapeutic dosage levels. A physician who consistently prescribes at levels much below those indicated is probably not treating his patients adequately.

Many physicians prescribe drugs at low dosages in their concern over side effects. While this concern is legitimate, the goal of treatment is symptomatic relief, and this will be less likely to occur if homeopathic (low) drug doses are used. It is ultimately far more satisfying for the physician, collaborating mental health workers, and the patient himself to experience relief from distressing symptoms (perhaps with some side effects), than for the patient to be treated for long periods of time with a variety of under-prescribed drugs to little or no therapeutic effect. Patients treated at low dosage levels, with no benefit, may become demoralized, feeling they are truly beyond help.

Side effects, when they appear, can be dealt with through reduction of dosage, drug change, or the use of adjunctive medication. Rarely will an effective drug have to be discontinued completely because of the appearance of toxic side effects, although this does occur.

INAPPROPRIATE DRUG TRIAL LENGTH

In addition to maintaining dose levels, it is necessary in drug trials to continue medication for a sufficient length of time to determine whether the drug is producing the desired effect. In most cases, treatment plans should include both a dosage build-up schedule, and a specified time period at the end of which therapeutic effects will be assessed. With antidepressants, a minimum trial period from 3 to 4 weeks, possibly up to 6 weeks, is necessary. If an antidepressant drug does not have effect within this time span, it is inappropriate to extend its use, in view of the prolonged suffering of the patient. A second drug, preferably of a different drug class, should then be tried.

A related error is the tendency to continue with a drug when there has been an only partial therapeutic response. Physicians have available several classes of drugs to try with each major diagnostic subgroup, so that if, for example, a schizophrenic's response to a specific phenothiazine does not seem favorable, there is little reason why a butyrophenone or thioxanthene should not be tried.

FAILURE TO OBSERVE DRUG "WASH-OUT" PERIODS

Because of possible toxic effects when switching between MAO inhibitors and tricyclic antidepressants, there should be a waiting period, usually 7–10 days, after stopping one type of drug and starting the other. Some researchers suggest that this may be ultraconservative, but until conclusively demonstrated to the contrary, the wash-out period is consistent with current concepts of good practice.

When taking on a patient previously treated elsewhere, the accompanying clinical case material is often vague; thus, the basis for prior diagnostic and treatment decisions may be quite unclear. If the patient has been receiving psychotropic drugs, the psychiatrist is faced with the decision of stopping or continuing the patient's existing drug program. Although one cannot make a single general rule to apply to all such cases, *when the patient's diagnostic status is unclear*, it does make sense to stop all medication during an initial evaluation period. This would mean that a patient with an unequivocal history of recurrent schizophrenia would remain on maintenance phenothiazines, just as the manic-depressive would remain on prophylactic lithium. But in most cases where there is diagnostic confusion, it is sensible to withdraw the patient from all medication in order to get a more accurate estimate of the patient's true clinical status. Special problems arise with character disorder patients, particularly hysterical patients who may have been inappropriately treated with phenothiazines. Since antipsychotic drugs can regularly be expected to make hysterical patients more symptomatic, the concurrent use of these drugs during the diagnostic evaluation serves both to exacerbate the condition and obscure the patient's diagnostic status.

TITRATING SYMPTOMATOLOGY

Another common therapeutic error is the tendency among some physicians to raise or lower dosage with every complaint reported by the patient. Since the effects of most psychotropic drugs are long lasting, it is much more sensible to set an overall treatment program for the patient; major changes should then be relatively infrequent, based only on significant changes in the patient's clinical condition.

The error of titrating symptomatology typically takes place at two stages in the patient's course, each time with potentially significant implications.

1. During the initial phase of treatment when the physician should be building up to therapeutic levels, he should avoid responding too quickly to minor improvements in the patient's condition. With premature leveling or decrease in drug dosage, modest gains may prove to be short-lived.

2. Perhaps an even more widespread and damaging possibility is the premature reduction or withdrawal of medication in patients for whom prophylactic drug use should be a significant part of the total treatment program. Many patients with chronic, recurrent disorders require maintenance medication to prevent relapse (as discussed in Chapter 9). However, this point is poorly understood by many physicians who come under pressure from patients who want to be free of the burden, expense, and onus of taking chronic medication. To many patients, medication is an unpleasant reminder of past problems, signifying that they require a "crutch," underscoring their inability to deal with their problems by themselves. The physician who bends too readily to the wishes of his patients to be free of medication is doing a disservice. It is far less

painful for an intact patient to deal in psychotherapy with his attitudes toward drug taking and the significance this has for him and his concept of self, than to attempt to pick up the pieces again after relapse.

REPEATED USE OF THE SAME DRUGS

Most psychiatrists who are well-trained in psychopharmacology develop some favorites among the major drug classes—drugs whose activity and proper dosage indications have become familiar. This is quite acceptable since there is usually little difference in the indications for various members of the same drug class. For good reasons, therefore, most psychiatrists are reluctant to prescribe drugs with whose action they are unfamiliar. This is a conservative practice, and one with probable benefits to the patient, since he is less likely to serve as a guinea pig for the physician. Therefore, the fact that a physician uses the same drugs repeatedly with different patients is not to be condemned, unless the choice of drug class or dosage is inappropriate for the patient.

INITIATING TWO DRUGS SIMULTANEOUSLY

Where diagnostic issues are unclear, and where the physician hopes to use drug response as a diagnostic aid, it is essential that the treatment picture be kept as "clean" as possible. If two psychoactive drugs are initiated at the same time, it is impossible to determine which of the two is responsible for subsequent clinical fluctuation. Therefore, psychoactive drugs should be introduced one at a time when drug response is to be used diagnostically.

FAILURE TO USE ANTIPARKINSON AGENTS

Once parkinson symptoms appear, antiparkinson agents should be prescribed promptly unless drug dosage reduction alone is effective, or unless there is a specific patient idiosyncracy (e.g., allergy). When the patient's treatment plan calls for relatively high doses of antipsychotics, there is little reason why the treating doctor should not concurrently prescribe antiparkinson agents. Detractors from this controversial issue point out that antiparkinson agents themselves produce side effects ranging from dry mouth to hallucinations, and caution against their routine use for prophylaxis.

Many clinicians fail to recognize certain side effects of antipsychotic drugs that can be mistaken for manifestations of the psychological disorder (e.g., akinesia is often mistaken for the psychomotor retardation of depression, and akathisia is easily misinterpreted as agitation). The use of prophylactic antiparkinson treatment concurrent with antipsychotic drugs reduces or eliminates these uncomfortable sources of diagnostic confusion.

Overuse of ECT

Related to the problem of drug choice is the indiscriminate use of ECT. In most areas, the local "shock mill" is known to all practitioners; referrals to such institutions should be avoided. This statement is not to be taken as a blanket condemnation of ECT. Where appropriate, ECT, with or without concurrent psychoactive drugs, may be a very useful treatment choice (see Chapter 7).

Medical Considerations

The good psychiatrist is first a good physician. He must take into account the patient's developmental status, general medical condition, and any specific physical problems. When the patient's physical condition is in doubt, the psychiatrist should not hesitate to refer to an internist or the family physician for appropriate evaluation.

Drugs are not generally prescribed in adult doses to pediatric, geriatric, or debilitated patients, or those with kidney or liver disease whose ability to detoxify the drug might be impaired. The risks of overdose are far greater in such patients and, therefore, drug selection as well as dosage levels must be chosen in light of the patient's developmental and medical status.

Failure to Perform Supporting Laboratory Work

As part of the initial medical evaluation of a patient, it may be desirable to perform special studies such as blood tests and electrocardiograms. Also important is the performance of routine laboratory work as part of certain treatment regimens. For example, because of the toxic risk and the possibility of therapeutic underdosage, it is essential to monitor the blood levels of patients taking lithium. The psychiatrist should ensure that appropriate laboratory studies are performed when indicated.

Periodic Reevaluation

Once a patient's condition has been stabilized, the physician may discontinue all drugs or place the patient on maintenance medication. The nonmedical collaborator then has a major responsibility to monitor the clinical status of such patients and refer them back to the physician when there are signs of deterioration. It is good practice for the physician to schedule follow-up interviews at regular intervals, perhaps every 3–6 months. The collaborating mental health worker should welcome this periodic review because it allows for consensual validation of one's own clinical impression of the patient; this is always in the patient's interest.

The Overdose Problem

In sufficiently large doses, many of the drugs discussed in this book can be fatal. This risk varies widely among different drug classes, and so the possibility of a potential overdose problem should always be kept in mind even if the patient is not currently suicidal. Thus, it may be advisable to have the patient refill his prescription often, rather than order him a long-term supply of drugs. The hazard in ordering drugs in large amounts with each prescription is particularly great with meprobamate, the barbiturates, and the MAO inhibitors. Several weeks' supply of these drugs in usual therapeutic doses, if taken at one time could be fatal. Therefore, one can seriously question the wisdom of psychotropic drugs being supplied to patients in large quantities, unless it is absolutely clear that the patient *and his family members* present no suicidal risk. Since it will frequently be impossible to make this determination, the most prudent course is to provide relatively small quantities of such medication with each prescription where there is any risk of suicide.

FAILURE TO COUNSEL PATIENTS ABOUT DRUG EFFECTS

The physician should always spend some time telling the patient about the projected treatment course. This generally helps allay anxieties, indicating to the patient what he can expect. Such counseling should include discussion of possible side effects, so that the patient is prepared should these occur. While this should be neither a frightening nor encyclopedic review of all possible reactions, the patient should nevertheless have some warning about possible side reactions. This is also a suitable time to discuss the need for any supporting laboratory studies, so that the patient does not suspect these signify some unusual medical condition. Moreover, any necessary precautions should be presented [e.g., referring a patient taking an MAO inhibitor to a list of restricted foods (see Appendix 6), or cautioning against drinking alcohol when taking certain drugs].

USE OF SOPORIFIC DRUGS DURING THE DAY

When soporific drugs (including the antipsychotics, antidepressants, and antianxiety agents) are prescribed, the total daily dose should usually be taken at the time of retiring, or in unequally divided daily doses with the largest dose at bedtime. Since all psychoactive drugs tend to be long-acting, and their sedative effects appear within an hour or two after oral ingestion, their general use at bedtime is to be encouraged. A significant exception is lithium which should always be prescribed in equal, divided doses to ensure relatively stable blood levels throughout the day.

FAILURE TO MONITOR PATIENT'S DRUG USE

It cannot be assumed that because medication is prescribed, the patient is taking it. Therefore, when there are major shifts in the patient's clinical state, an immediate question is whether the patient has been taking the prescribed medication. Where necessary, the physician should not be reluctant to have urine tests performed in order to determine whether or not the patient has actually been taking his drugs. Possible solutions to the problem of a patient's failure to take prescribed drugs include:

1. Encouraging the family to assume greater responsibility in overseeing medication taking.
2. Use of liquid medication which cannot easily be "cheeked," as is frequently done to avoid swallowing tablets or capsules.
3. Use of fluphenazine enanthate, fluphenazine decanoate, or other long-acting, injectable preparations.

ABRUPT WITHDRAWAL

The use of all psychotropic medication involves some physiological habituation, so that some degree of withdrawal symptoms is expected with abrupt discontinuation. Minor withdrawal symptoms can include malaise, nausea, headache, or diarrhea, while serious withdrawal symptoms such as seizures, are also possible. Therefore, as a routine practice, drug discontinuation should be gradual rather than abrupt, as a means of minimizing patient discomfort at this point in treatment.

Misuse of Antipsychotic Agents in Anxiety States

A common therapeutic error is the use of antipsychotic agents in low dosages for the treatment of simple, anticipatory anxiety states. As noted in Chapter 3, this may be countertherapeutic in certain classes of patients (for example, hysterical character disorders).

Misuse of Minor Tranquilizers for Panic Attacks

Antidepressants are specifically indicated in panic attacks. A very common therapeutic error is the treatment of phobic-anxious patients with antipsychotic or antianxiety agents. The appropriate use of an antidepressant for acute anxiety attacks with a concurrent antianxiety agent targeted for associated anticipatory anxiety has been detailed in Chapter 2.

Overuse of Amphetamines

Because the hazards of amphetamine use are great and the therapeutic indications almost nonexistent (except for hyperactive children) prescription of stimulants should be rare. One should seriously question (*a*) prolonged amphetamine use in any psychiatric patient, and (*b*) prescription of amphetamines to a significant proportion of a psychiatrist's patients.

Overview

Mastery of the material in this book will probably place the reader at a level of psychopharmacologic sophistication greater than that of many members of the medical community. With the guidelines provided in this chapter, the level of a colleague's psychotropic drug practice may be better evaluated. In discussing a joint therapeutic problem, the physician should be able to describe a sensible rationale for his chemotherapeutic program. If he cannot, he is himself probably confused about the case.

The price of psychopharmacologic sophistication is professional role diffusion and conflict. The psychiatrist who has been accustomed to regarding himself as the "head" of the treatment team or certainly as that colleague most knowledgeable about such medical matters as drug treatment, now finds himself challenged by some upstart from outside the medical "fraternity." How can this situation be handled?

First, bear in mind that the psychiatric field in general is experiencing growing pains, not simply in the area of psychopharmacology. Nursing personnel are diagnosing cases and making treatment plans, psychologists are running wards, physicians are doing behavior therapy, social workers are doing individual psychotherapy. The old role models are all breaking down, making everyone a bit uncomfortable; this hopefully indicates progress in the field. Professional jealousies aside, from the patient's point of view it must be to his advantage to be treated by more knowledgeable personnel of whatever discipline.

Free and open case discussion of psychopharmacologic practice is always in the patient's interest, introducing an element of accountability into drug practice as the physician realizes his performance is being critically evaluated by his professional colleagues.

Be diplomatic. Remember that frontal attacks on a colleague's weak spots are rarely productive of positive change. Remember, too, that reading this book does not *ipso facto* qualify anyone as a psychopharmacologist.

CHAPTER 15

TRAINING IMPLICATIONS

We have tried to show that rational, psychopharmacologic treatment recommendations should be based on careful diagnostic evaluations. Before the development of effective psychopharmacologic treatment methods, diagnosis was unpopular and regarded by many mental health professionals as an academic exercise only. Now, diagnosis is again becoming an essential part of case management and clinical training. As the roles of new treatment methods such as psychopharmacology, individual behavior modification, and group treatment become recognized in psychiatry, psychology, social work, psychiatric nursing, occupational therapy, and related mental health disciplines, it is expected that there will be renewed interest in the differential diagnostic process as it relates to proper treatment choice.

It has become fashionable to attack the "medical model." In particular, three related concepts have come under attack:

1. Mental "illness" is felt by some to be an inappropriate way to describe an individual's problems in living.

2. "Diagnosis" is regarded as an archaic medical concept which does not harmonize with efforts to understand each client as a unique being.
3. Physical treatments are regarded as inappropriate methods of changing an individual's maladaptive habit patterns, serving only to deaden the client's awareness of his difficulties.

In stressing the social and interpersonal determinants of psychopathology, significant clinical research findings in psychopharmacology have often been ignored [e.g., Balance, Hirschfield and Bringmann (1970) and Sharma (1970)]. We share with others in the mental health field a concern for developing better models of psychopathology, but feel that there is still a good deal of potential value in the "medical model," particularly the use of careful diagnostic processes in the selection of appropriate treatment choices.

Disturbed behavior may result from a variety of known, presumed, or unknown causes. For example, visual hallucinations may result from alcohol or drug intoxication, lead poisoning, endocrinological disease, as well as supposed "functional" or hysterical mechanisms. These distinctions are important because there are now a variety of therapeutic techniques available, and no single therapist is expert in all types of treatment (e.g., desensitization, relearning therapies, psychoanalysis, drugs, and milieu manipulation). Each patient's therapeutic needs should be evaluated individually, and referrals made where necessary. Before the present era of therapeutic specialization, it was generally assumed that either psychoanalytic or Rogerian psychotherapy was the treatment of choice for all mental illness. Then, the arguments against patient classification may have been justified. Now, with a broader range of therapeutic possibilities, the problems of differential diagnosis and treatment prescription are much more important (especially when measured in terms of a patient's suffering before an effective treatment strategy is devised). To provide optimal treatment, one has to specify as clearly as possible the conditions for which treatment is sought. In this context, diagnosis can serve a useful function both in making rational treatment recommendations and in helping to understand the likely prognosis of untreated cases.

Concerning prognosis, many mental health workers seem to have adopted a professional ethic which says, "Let us regard each person who comes for treatment as having an equal chance of success." Longitudinal studies of patients in a variety of diagnostic groups show that this blanket optimism is unwarranted. One might argue, nonetheless, that as a treatment strategy, it is useful to behave *as though* each patient had an equally good chance of favorable response to treatment. While this strategy may have some merit, it should not blind us to the fact that different psychopathologic states do have different expected outcomes. For example, untreated manic-depressive patients can be expected to have a lifelong pattern of mood disregulation, with relatively normal periods of remission. Cyclic schizophrenic patients, on the other hand, generally exhibit deteriorating trends, so that with repeated episodes there is increased functional impairment.

Like the time-honored efforts of taxonomists in all areas of science, contemporary taxonomists in the field of psychopathology are trying to make sense of a seemingly chaotic set of phenomena. Toward this end there is now a respectable and growing body of research aimed at improving classification methods in a variety of ways (Katz *et al.*, 1968).

About general medicine it has been said, "A diagnosis is of value in indicating the etiology, . . . treatment, and prognosis of disease" (Sharma, 1970, p. 251). The results of recent clinical research indicate that these are desirable goals in psychological disturbance as well. The utility or nonutility of diagnostic methods in psychiatry should be evaluated against these very criteria. That is, unless classification methods can be shown to be valid (having etiologic, therapeutic, or predictive value), then they are merely academic exercises with no practical use.

Psychopharmacology research of the 1960s leads one to conclude that there are diagnosis–drug interactions. For many psychiatric conditions, drug treatment is significantly superior to placebo. Beyond that, it is now established that certain drugs have a higher likelihood of success in specific classes of patients. Sophisticated work in clinical psychopharmacology is concerned no longer with simply establishing overall drug efficacy, but rather with selecting the right drug for the right patient (Klein, 1967; Klett and Moseley, 1965).

Based on a series of original investigations, as well as an extensive literature review, Klein and Davis (1969) concluded that suitably modified diagnoses do provide a useful way of classifying patients for (a) making prognostic statements about expected long-term outcomes, and (b) making more rational, specific treatment recommendations.

Some patients whose behavior pathology seems to reflect disturbed social learning respond very favorably to chemotherapy. Phobic-anxiety reactions (seen in early life as school phobia or in later life as serious separation-anxiety) seem to fit an interpersonal model of etiology. Surprisingly, many such patients respond well to antidepressants. Because these psychopathologic conditions can be readily interpreted as due to faulty social learning, a practitioner unfamiliar with drug therapy might fail to make an appropriate referral simply through ignorance. Similarly, medical practitioners can mishandle cases through the sole use of drugs, where psychotherapy or other nondrug approaches may be the primary or secondary treatment choice. Optimal treatment, from the patient's point of view, obviously requires cooperation and mutual respect by all mental health workers, particulary in this era of ever greater therapeutic specialization.

As discussed throughout this book, there are now more or less clearly established indications and contraindications for a wide range of drugs in the treatment of a variety of psychotic, affective, and personality disorders. The most useful way of organizing this information seems to be a modification of the standard diagnostic nomenclature. Research aimed at objectifying the psychiatric diagnostic process is reported with increased frequency (e.g., Honigfeld *et al.*, 1969; Lusted and Stahl, 1969; Nathan, 1967, Spitzer and Endicott, 1968).

Until current information on diagnosis and drug treatment is made more generally available in professional training programs, the current level of mental health care in the United States will remain inadequate.

ALPHABETICAL LIST OF GENERIC DRUG NAMES, WITH TRADE NAMES, MANUFACTURER, AND DRUG TYPE

Generic name	Trade name	Manufacturer	Drug type
Acetophenazine	Tindal	Schering	Antipsychotic
Acepromazine	Notensil, Plegicil	Clin-Byla	Antipsychotic
Acetylcarbromal	Sedamyl	Riker	Sedative
Amitriptyline	Elavil	Merck, Sharp & Dohme	Antidepressant
Amobarbital	Amytal	Lilly	Sedative
Amphetamine	Benzedrine	Smith, Kline & French	Stimulant
Azacyclonol	Frenquel	Merrell	Antianxiety
Benactyzine	Suavitil	Merck, Sharp & Dohme	Antianxiety
Benzphetamine	Didrex	Upjohn	Stimulant
Benzquinamide	Quantril	Pfizer	Antianxiety
Benztropine	Cogentin	Merck, Sharp & Dohme	Antiparkinson

Generic name	Trade name	Manufacturer	Drug type
Biperiden	Akineton	Knoll	Antiparkinson
Bromisovalum	Bromural	Knoll	Antianxiety
Butabarbital	Butisol	McNeil	Sedative
Butaperazine	Repoise	A. H. Robins	Antipsychotic
Captodiame	Suvren	Ayerst	Antianxiety
Carbamazepine	Tegretol	Geigy	Antidepressant
Carphenazine	Proketazine	Wyeth	Antipsychotic
Chloral betaine	Beta-Chlor	Mead Johnson	Sedative
Chloral hydrate	Felsules	Fellows-Testagar	Sedative
	Kessodrate	McKesson	
	Noctec	Squibb	
	Somnos	Merck, Sharp & Dohme	
Chlordiazepoxide	Librium	Roche	Antianxiety
Chlormethazanone	Trancopal	Sterling-Winthrop	Antianxiety
Chlorpromazine	Largactil	Rhone-Poulenc	Antipsychotic
	Thorazine	Smith, Kline & French	
Chlorprothixene	Taractan	Roche	Antianxiety
Cyclazocine		Sterling-Winthrop	Heroin antagonist
Deanol	Deaner	Riker	Stimulant
Desipramine	Norpramin	Lakeside	Antidepressant
	Pertofrane	Geigy	
Dextroamphetamine	Dexedrine	Smith, Kline & French	Stimulant
	Dexaspan	USV Pharmaceutical	
	Dexa-Sequels	Lederle	
	PERKē ONE	Ascher	
Dextroamphetamine tannate	Obotan	Mallinckrodt	Stimulant
Diazepam	Valium	Roche	Antianxiety
Diphenylhydantoin	Toin	Reid Provident	Anticonvulsant
	Ekko	Fleming	
	Dilantin	Parke-Davis	
	Kessodanten	McKesson	

Generic name	Trade name	Manufacturer	Drug type
Disulfiram	Antabuse	Ayerst	Alcohol antagonist
Doxepin	Sinequan	Pfizer	Antidepressant
Ethosuximide	Zarontin	Parke-Davis	Anticonvulsant
Ethinamate	Valmid	Lilly	Hypnotic
Ethchlorvynol	Placidyl	Abbott	Hypnotic
Ethotoin	Peganone	Abbott	Anticonvulsant
Fluphenazine	Prolixin Permitil	Squibb Schering	Antipsychotic
Flurazepam	Dalmane	Roche	Hypnotic
Glutethimide	Doriden	Ciba	Hypnotic
Haloperidol	Haldol Serenace	McNeil Searle	Antipsychotic
Heptabarbital	Medomin	Geigy	Sedative
Hydroxyzine	Atarax Vistaril	Roering Pfizer	Antianxiety
Hydroxyphenamate	Listica	Armour	Antianxiety
Imipramine	Tofranil	Smith, Kline & French	Antimanic
Isocarboxazid	Marplan	Roche	Antidepressant
Levamphetamine	Amodril	North American Pharmacal	Stimulant
	Cydril	Tutag	
	Pedestal	Len-Tag	
Lithium	Eskalith	Smith, Kline & French	Antimanic
	Lithonate	Rowell	
	Lithane	Roerig	
Mepazine	Pacatal	Warner-Chilcott	Antipsychotic
Mephanoxalone	Trepidone	Lederle	Antianxiety
Mephobarbital	Mebaral	Winthrop	Anticonvulsant
Meprobamate	Kesso-bamate Equanil Miltown	McKesson Wyeth Wallace	Antianxiety
Mesoridazine	Serentil	Sandoz	Antipsychotic

Generic name	Trade name	Manufacturer	Drug type
Methamphetamine	Amphedroxyn	Lilly	Stimulant
	Desoxyn	Abbott	
Methadone	Dolophine	Lilly	Heroin substitute
Methaqualone	Quaalude	Wm. H. Rorer	Hypnotic
	Parest	Parke-Davis	
	Sopor	Arnar-Stone	
	Somnafac	Smith, Miller, Patch	
Metharbital	Gemonil	Abbott	Sedative
Methoxypromazine	Tentone	Lederle	Antianxiety
Methsuximide	Celontin	Parke-Davis	Anticonvulsant
Methylpentynol	Dormison	Schering	Hypnotic
Methylphenidate	Ritalin	Ciba	Stimulant
Methyprylon	Noludar	Roche	Hypnotic
Methysergide	Sansert	Sandoz	
Nalaxone	Narcan	Endo	Heroin antagonist
Nalorphine	Lethidrone	Burroughs-Wellcome	Heroin substitute
	Nalline	Merck	
Nialamide	Niamid	Pfizer	Antidepressant
Nortriptyline	Aventyl	Lilly	Antidepressant
Opipramol	Ensidon	Geigy	Antidepressant
Oxanamide	Quiactin	Merrell	Antianxiety
Oxazepam	Serax	Wyeth	Antianxiety
Paraldehyde	Paral	Fellows-Testagar	Sedative
Pargyline	Eutonyl	Abbott	Antidepressant
Pentobarbital	Nembutal	Abbott	Sedative
	Pentobarbital	Lilly	
Pentylenetetrazol	Nioric	Ascher	Stimulant
	Metrazol	Knoll	
Perphenazine	Trilafon	Schering	Antipsychotic
Phenacemide	Phenurone	Abbott	Anticonvulsant
Phenaglycodol	Ultran	Lilly	Antianxiety
Phenelzine	Nardil	Warner-Chilcott	Antidepressant
Phenmetrazine	Preludin	Geigy	Stimulant

Generic name	Trade name	Manufacturer	Drug type
Phenobarbital	Eskabarb	Smith, Kline & French	Sedative
	Luminal	Winthrop	
	Phenobarbital	Lilly	
	Stental	A. H. Robins	
Phensuximide	Milontin	Parke-Davis	Anticonvulsant
Pipamazine	Mornidine	Searle	Antipsychotic
Piperacetazine	Quide	Dow	Antipsychotic
Primidone	Mysoline	Ayerst	Anticonvulsant
Prochlorperazine	Compazine	Smith, Kline & French	Antipsychotic
Procyclidine	Kemadrin	Burroughs-Wellcome	Antiparkinson
Promazine	Sparine	Wyeth	Antipsychotic
Promethazine	Phenergan	Wyeth	Antipsychotic
Propericiazine	Neuleptil	Rhone-Poulenc	Antipsychotic
Protriptyline	Vivactil	Merck, Sharp & Dohme	Antidepressant
Secobarbital	Seconal	Lilly	Sedative
Talbutal	Lotusate	Winthrop	Sedative
Thiethylperazine	Torecan	Sandoz	Antipsychotic
Thiopropazate	Dartal	Searle	Antipsychotic
Thioproperazine	Majeptil	Rhone-Poulenc	Antipsychotic
Thioridazine	Mellaril	Sandoz	Antipsychotic
Thiothixene	Navane	Roerig	Antipsychotic
Tranylcypromine	Parnate	Smith, Kline & French	Antidepressant
Trifluoperazine	Stelazine	Smith, Kline & French	Antipsychotic
Triflupromazine	Vesprin	Squibb	Antipsychotic
Trihexyphenidyl	Artane	Lederle	Antiparkinson
Trimethadione	Tridione	Abbott	Anticonvulsant
Trimipramine	Surmontil	Rhone-Poulenc	Antidepressant
Tybamate	Solacen	Wallace	Antianxiety
	Tybatran	A. H. Robins	

ALPHABETICAL LIST OF DRUG TRADE NAMES, CHEMICAL COMPOSITION, MANUFACTURER, AND DRUG TYPE

Trade name	Chemical composition	Manufacturer	Drug type[a]
Actomol	mebanazine	Imperial Chemical Industry	Antidepressant
Adipex	methamphetamine amobarbital	Lemmon	
Akineton	biperiden	Knoll	Antiparkinson
Amodex	dextroamphetamine amobarbital	Fellows-Testagar	
Amodril	levamphetamine	North American Pharmacal	Stimulant
Amphaplex	methamphetamine saccharate methamphetamine hydrochloride amphetamine dextroamphetamine	Palmedico	Stimulant

[a] Drug type not indicated for combination drugs.

Trade name	Chemical composition	Manufacturer	Drug type[a]
Amphedroxyn	methamphetamine	Lilly	Stimulant
Amphodex	dextroamphetamine amorbital vitamins	Jamieson-McKames	
Amytal	amobarbital	Lilly	Sedative
Antabuse	disulfiram	Ayerst	Alcohol antagonist
Artane	trihexyphenidyl	Lederle	Antiparkinson
Atarax	hydroxyzine	Roerig	Antianxiety
Aventyl	nortriptyline	Lilly	Antidepressant
Bamadex	dextroamphetamine	Lederle	
Benizol	pentylenetetrazol nicotinic acid	Bentex	Stimulant
Benzedrine	amphetamine	Smith, Kline & French	Stimulant
Beta-chlor	chloral betaine	Mead-Johnson	Sedative
Biphetamine	dextroamphetamine amphetamine methaqualone	Strasenburgh	
Bromural	bromisovalum	Knoll	Antianxiety
Butatrax	amobarbital butabarbital	Sutliff & Case	Sedative
Butisol	butabarbital	McNeil	Sedative
Carbrital	pentobarbital carbromal	Parke-Davis	Sedative
Celontin	methsuximide	Parke-Davis	Anticonvulsant
Cogentin	benztropine	Merck, Sharp & Dohme	Antiparkinson
Compazine	prochlorperazine	Smith, Kline & French	Antianxiety
Cyclazocine	cyclazocine	Sterling-Winthrop	Heroin antagonist
Dalmane	flurazepam	Roche	Hypnotic
Dartal	thiopropazate	Searle	Antipsychotic
Deaner	deanol	Riker	Stimulant
Deprol	meprobamate benactyzine	Wallace	

Trade name	Chemical composition	Manufacturer	Drug type[a]
Desbutal	methamphetamine pentobarbital	Abbott	
Desoxyn	methamphetamine	Abbott	Stimulant
Dexamyl	dextroamphetamine amobarbital	Smith, Kline & French	
Dexa-Sequels	dextroamphetamine	Lederle	Stimulant
Dexaspan	dextroamphetamine	USV Pharmaceutical	Stimulant
Dexedrine	dextroamphetamine	Smith, Kline & French	Stimulant
Didrex	benzphetamine	Upjohn	Stimulant
Dilantin	diphenylhydantoin	Parke-Davis	Anticonvulsant
Di-phenyl	diphenylhydantoin	Drug Industries	Anticonvulsant
Dolophine	methadone	Lilly	Heroin substitute
Doriden	glutethimide	Ciba	Hypnotic
Dormison	methylpentynol	Schering	Hypnotic
Ekko	diphenylhydantoin	Fleming	Anticonvulsant
Elavil	amitriptyline	Merck, Sharp & Dohme	Antidepressant
Ensidon	opipramol	Geigy	Antidepressant
Equanil	meprobamate	Wyeth	Antianxiety
Eskabarb	phenobarbital	Smith, Kline & French	Sedative
Eskalith	lithium	Smith, Kline & French	Antimanic
Eskaphen B	phenobarbital thiamine	Smith, Kline & French	
Etrafon	perphenazine amitriptyline	Schering	
Eutonyl	pargyline	Abbott	Antidepressant
Felsules	chloral hydrate	Fellows-Testagar	Sedative
Frenquel	azacyclonol	Merrell	Antianxiety
Gemonil	metharbital	Abbott	Sedative
Haldol	haloperidol	McNeil	Antipsychotic
Kemadrin	procyclidine	Burroughs-Wellcome	Antiparkinson

Trade name	Chemical composition	Manufacturer	Drug type[a]
Kesso-Bamate	meprobamate	McKesson	Antianxiety
Kessodanten	diphenylhydantoin	McKesson	Anticonvulsant
Kessodrate	chloral hydrate	McKesson	Sedative
Largactil	chlorpromazine	Rhone-Poulenc	Antipsychotic
Lethidrone	nalorphine	Burroughs-Wellcome	Heroin substitute
Librium	chlordiazepoxide	Roche	Antianxiety
Listica	hydroxyphenamate	Armour	Antianxiety
Lithane	lithium	Roerig	Antimanic
Lithonate	lithium	Rowell	Antimanic
Lotusate	talbutal	Winthrop	Sedative
Luminal	phenobarbital	Winthrop	Sedative
Majeptil	thioproperazine	Rhone-Poulenc	Antipsychotic
Marplan	isocarboxazid	Roche	Antidepressant
Mebaral	mephobarbital	Winthrop	Sedative
Mebroin	mephobarbital diphenylhydantoin	Winthrop	Anticonvulsant
Medomin	heptabarbital	Geigy	Sedative
Mellaril	thioridazine	Sandoz	Antipsychotic
Meprospan	meprobamate	Wallace	Antianxiety
Mesantoin	mephenytoin	Sandoz	Anticonvulsant
Methadone	methadone	CRW	Heroin substitute
Methedrine	methamphetamine	Burroughs-Wellcome	Stimulant
Metrazol	pentylenetetrazol	Knoll	Stimulant
Milontin	phensuximide	Parke-Davis	Anticonvulsant
Miltown	meprobamate	Wallace	Antianxiety
Mornidine	pipamazine	Searle	Antipsychotic
Mysoline	primidone	Ayerst	Anticonvulsant
Nalline	nalorphine	Merck, Sharp & Dohme	Heroin substitute
Narcan	nalaxone	Endo	Heroin antagonist
Nardil	phenelzine	Warner-Chilcott	Antidepressant

Trade name	Chemical composition	Manufacturer	Drug type[a]
Navane	thiothixene	Roerig	Antipsychotic
Nembutal	pentobarbital	Abbott	Sedative
Neuleptil	propericiazine	Rhone-Poulenc	Antipsychotic
Niamid	nialamide	Pfizer	Antidepressant
Nioric	pentylenetetrazol	Ascher	Stimulant
Noctec	chloral hydrate	Squibb	Sedative
Noludar	methyprylon	Roche	Hypnotic
Norpramin	desipramine	Lakeside	Antidepressant
Obedrin	methamphetamine pentobarbital	Semed	
Obetrol	methamphetamine saccharate methamphetamine hydrochloride amphetamine sulfate dextroamphetamine	Obetrol	
Obotan	dextroamphetamine tannate	Mallinckrodt	Stimulant
Obotan-S	dextroamphetamine tannate secobarbital	Mallinckrodt	
Olbese No. 1	amobarbital methamphetamine	Drug Industries	
Pacatal	mepazine	Warner-Chilcott	Antipsychotic
Paradione	paramethadione	Abbott	Anticonvulsant
Paral	paraldehyde	Fellows-Testagar	Sedative
Parest	methaqualone	Parke-Davis	Hypnotic
Parnate	tranylcypromine	Smith, Kline & French	Antidepressant
Pedestal	levo-amphetamine succinate	Len-Tag	Stimulant
Peganone	ethotoin	Abbott	Anticonvulsant
Penotal	phenobarbital pentobarbital	Coastal	Sedative
Pentobarbital	pentobarbital	Lilly	Sedative

Trade name	Chemical composition	Manufacturer	Drug type[a]
PERKē ONE	dextroamphetamine	Ascher	Stimulant
PERKē TWO	dextroamphetamine amobarbital	Ascher	
Permitil	fluphenazine	Schering	Antipsychotic
Pertofrane	desipramine	Geigy	Antidepressant
Phelantin	diphenylhydantoin phenobarbital methamphetamine	Parke-Davis	Anticonvulsant
Phenergan	promethazine	Wyeth	Antipsychotic
Phenobarbital	phenobarbital	Lilly	Sedative
Phenurone	phenacemide	Abbott	Anticonvulsant
Placidyl	ethchlorvynol	Abbott	Hypnotic
Plexonal	diethylbarbiturate phenylethylbarbiturate isobutylallylbarbital scopolamine dihydroergotamine methanesulfate	Sandoz	
Preludin	phenmetrazine	Geigy	Stimulant
Proketazine	carphenazine	Wyeth	Antipsychotic
Prolixin	fluphenazine	Squibb	Antipsychotic
Providex	dextroamphetamine amobarbital	Reid-Provident	
Quaalude	methaqualone	Wm. H. Rorer	Hypnotic
Quadamine	dextroamphetamine amobarbital vitamins	Len-Tag	
Quantril	benzquinamide	Pfizer	Antianxiety
Quiactin	oxanamide	Merrell	Antianxiety
Quide	piperacetazine	Dow	Antipsychotic
Repoise	butaperazine	A. H. Robins	Antipsychotic
Ritalin	methylphenidate	Ciba	Stimulant
Sansert	methysergide	Sandoz	Experimental
Seconal	secobarbital	Lilly	Sedative
Sedamyl	acetylcarbromal	Riker	Sedative

Trade name	Chemical composition	Manufacturer	Drug type[a]
Serax	oxazepam	Wyeth	Antianxiety
Serenace	haloperidol	Searle	Antipsychotic
Serentil	mesoridazine	Sandoz	Antipsychotic
Sinequan	doxepin	Pfizer	Antidepressant
Softran	buclizine	Stuart	Antianxiety
Solacen	tybamate	Wallace	Antianxiety
Somnafac	methaqualone	Smith, Miller & Patch	Hypnotic
Somnos	chloral hydrate	Merck, Sharp & Dohme	Sedative
Sopor	methaqualone	Arnar-Stone	Hypnotic
Sparine	promazine	Wyeth	Antipsychotic
Stelazine	trifluoperazine	Smith, Kline & French	Antipsychotic
Stental	phenobarbital	A. H. Robins	Sedative
Suavitil	benactyzine	Merck, Sharp & Dohme	Antianxiety
Surmontil	trimipramine	Rhone-Poulenc	Antidepressant
Taractan	chlorprothixene	Roche	Antipsychotic
Tegretol	carbamazepine	Geigy	Antidepressant
Tentone	methoxypromazine	Lederle	Antianxiety
Thorazine	chlorpromazine	Smith, Kline & French	Antipsychotic
Tindal	acetophenazine	Schering	Antipsychotic
Tofranil	imipramine	Geigy	Antidepressant
Toin	diphenylhydantoin	Reid-Provident	Anticonvulsant
Torecan	thiethylperazine	Sandoz	Antipsychotic
Trancopal	chlormethazanone	Winthrop	Antianxiety
Trepidone	mephenoxalone	Lederle	Antianxiety
Triavil	perphenazine amitriptyline	Merck, Sharp & Dohme	
Tri-barbs	secobarbital butabarbital phenobarbital	High Chemical	Sedative

Trade name	Chemical composition	Manufacturer	Drug type[a]
Tridione	trimethadione	Abbott	Anticonvulsant
Trilafon	perphenazine	Schering	Antipsychotic
Tuinal	secobarbital amobarbital	Lilly	Sedative
Tybatran	tybamate	A. H. Robins	Antianxiety
Ultran	phenaglycodol	Lilly	Antianxiety
Valium	diazepam	Roche	Antianxiety
Valmid	ethinamate	Lilly	Hypnotic
Vesprin	triflupromazine	Squibb	Antipsychotic
Vibazine	buclizine	Pfizer	Antianxiety
Vistaril	hydroxyzine	Pfizer	Antianxiety
Vivactil	protriptyline	Merck, Sharp & Dohme	Antidepressant
Zarontin	ethosuximide	Parke-Davis	Anticonvulsant

PRODUCT IDENTIFICATION CHART BY TRADE NAME, SHOWING FORM, SHAPE, COLOR, AND SPECIFIC IDENTIFYING MARKS

Trade name	Chemical composition	Dosage (mg)	Form	Shape	Color	Special marks
Adipex	methamphetamine amobarbital	10 50	Capsule		Blue/white	
Adipex Ty-Med	methamphetamine amobarbital	10 50	Tablet	Round	Blue/white	
Akineton	biperiden	2	Tablet	Round (scored)	White	Knoll™
Amodex Jr.	dextroamphetamine amobarbital	7.5 30	Capsule	Capsule-shaped	Red/yellow	Fellows Testagar™ 045
Amodex	dextroamphetamine amobarbital	15 60	Capsule	Capsule-shaped	Brown/yellow	Fellows Testagar™ 050
Amodril	levamphetamine	21	Capsule	Capsule-shaped	Green/clear (Green/white pellets)	NAP
Amphaplex 10	methamphetamine saccharate methamphetamine amphetamine sulfate dextroamphetamine sulfate	2.5 2.5 2.5 2.5	Tablet	Round (scored)	Pink	Palmedico™
Amphaplex 20	methamphetamine saccharate methamphetamine amphetamine sulfate dextroamphetamine sulfate	5 5 5 5	Tablet	Round	Olive green	Palmedico™

Brand	Generic	Strength	Form	Shape	Color	Code
Amytal	amobarbital	15	Tablet	Flat, oblong (scored)	Green, light	Lilly™ T40
		30			Yellow	Lilly™ T56
		50			Orange	Lilly™ T37
		100			Pink	Lilly™ T32
Amytal	sodium amobarbital	65	Capsule		Blue	Lilly™ F23
		200				Lilly™ F33
Antabuse	disulfiram	250	Tablet	Round (scored)	White	Ayerst 809
		500				Ayerst 810
Artane	trihexyphenidyl	2	Tablet	Round (scored)	White	
		5	Tablet	Round (scored)	White	
Atarax	hydroxyzine	5	Capsule	Ovoid	Blue	Lederle™
		10	Tablet	Round	Orange	560
		25	Tablet	Round	Green	561
		50	Tablet	Round	Yellow	562
		100	Tablet	Round	Red	563
Aventyl	nortriptyline	10	Capsule		White/yellow	Lilly™ H17
		25				Lilly™ H19
Bamadex	dextroamphetamine meprobamate	5 400	Tablet	Round	Pink	
Bamadex sequels	dextroamphetamine meprobamate	15 300	Capsule		Orange (two-tone)	Lederle™
Benzedrine	amphetamine sulfate	5	Tablet	Triangular (scored)	Pink	A91
		10	Tablet	Triangular (scored)	Pink	A92
		15	Capsule		Purple/clear (pink/white pellets)	SKF A90

Trade name	Chemical composition	Dosage (mg)	Form	Shape	Color	Special marks
Beta-chlor	chloral betaine	870	Tablet	Oval	Pink (mottled)	Mead Johnson[TM] (MJ)
Biphetamine	dextroamphetamine amphetamine	3.75 3.75	Capsule		White	Strasenburgh[TM] 18–895
	dextroamphetamine amphetamine	6.25 6.25	Capsule		Black/white	Strasenburgh[TM] 18–878
	dextroamphetamine amphetamine	10 10	Capsule		Black	Strasenburgh[TM] 18–875
Biphetamine-T	dextroamphetamine amphetamine methaqualone	6.25 6.25 40	Capsule		Black/green	Strasenburgh[TM] 18–899
	dextroamphetamine amphetamine methaqualone	10 10 40	Capsule		Red/black	Strasenburgh[TM] 18–898
Bromural	bromisovalum	325	Tablet	Round	White	Knoll[TM]
Butatrax	amobarbital butabarbital	20 30	Capsule		Green/white	
Buticaps	sodium butabarbital	15 30 50 100	Capsule Capsule Capsule Capsule		Lavender/white Green/white Orange/white Pink/white	McNEIL McNEIL McNEIL McNEIL
Butisol	butabarbital	15 30 100	Tablet Tablet Tablet Tablet	Round (scored)	Lavender Green Orange Pink	McNEIL McNEIL McNEIL McNEIL

Brand	Generic	mg	Form	Shape	Color	Code
Butisol R-A	butabarbital	30	Tablet	Round	White	McNEIL (in lavender)
		60	Tablet	Round	White	McNEIL (in green)
Carbrital	pentobarbital sodium carbromal	97.5 260	Capsule	Round	White, blue band	P-D 376
	pentobarbital sodium carbromal	48.5 130	Capsule	Round	White, blue band	P-D 372
Celontin	methsuximide	150	Capsule		Yellow, brown band	P-D 537
		300	Capsule		Yellow, orange band	P-D 525
Cogentin	benztropine mesylate	0.5	Tablet	Round (scored)	White	MSD 21
		1	Tablet	Oval (scored)	White	MSD 635
		2	Tablet	Round (cross scored)	White	MSD 60
Compazine	prochlorperazine	5	Tablet	Round	Yellow	SKF 5 C66
		10	Tablet	Round	Yellow	SKF 10 C67
		25	Tablet	Round	Yellow	SKF 25 C69
Compazine Spansule	prochlorperazine	10	Capsule		Black/clear, (yellow/white pellets)	SKF (1 dot) C44
		15	Capsule			SKF (2 dots) C46
		30	Capsule			SKF (3 dots) C47
		75	Capsule			SKF (4 dots) C49
Cydril	levamphetamine succinate	7	Tablet	Round (scored)	Blue	TUTAG
		21	Capsule		Green/clear, dark green band (yellow/green pellets)	TUTAG

Trade name	Chemical composition	Dosage (mg)	Form	Shape	Color	Special marks
Dalmane	flurazepam	15	Capsule		Orange/ivory	ROCHE 65
		30	Capsule		Red/ivory	ROCHE 66
Dartal	thiopropazate	2	Tablet	Round	Red	Searle
		5	Tablet	Round	Red	Searle
		5	Tablet	Round	White	Searle
		10	Tablet	Round	Red	Searle
Deaner	deanol	25	Tablet	Round (scored)	White	RIKER
		100	Tablet	Round (scored)	Pink	RIKER
Deprol	meprobamate benactyzine	400 1	Tablet	Round (scored)	Pink	Wallace[TM]
Desbutal	methamphetamine pentobarbital	5 30	Capsule		Green	Abbott[TM]
Desbutal Gradumet	methamphetamine sodium pentobarbital	10 60	Tablet	Round	Orange/blue	Abbott[TM]
	methamphetamine sodium pentobarbital	15 90	Tablet	Round	Yellow/blue	Abbott[TM]
Desoxyn	methamphetamine	2.5 5	Tablet Tablet	Round Round	White White	Abbott[TM]
Desoxyn Gradumet	methamphetamine	5 10 15	Tablet Tablet Tablet	Round Round Round	White Orange Yellow	Abbott[TM] Abbott[TM] Abbott[TM]
Dexamyl	dextroamphetamine amobarbital	5 32	Tablet	Triangular (scored)	Green	SKF D93

Name	Drug	Dosage	Form	Description	Code
Dexamyl Spansule	dextroamphetamine amobarbital	10 65	Capsule	Green/clear, (green/white pellets)	SKF D91 (1 dot)
	dextroamphetamine amobarbital	15 97	Capsule	Orange	SKF D92 (2 dots)
Dexa-Sequels	dextroamphetamine	10 15	Capsule Capsule	Ovoid Ovoid	Orange Orange	Lederle™ 10 mg Lederle™ 15 mg
Dexaspan	dextroamphetamine	15	Capsule		Orange/yellow	USV™
Dexaspan-B	dextroamphetamine amobarbital	15 100	Capsule		Yellow/green	USV™
Dexedrine	dextroamphetamine	5	Tablet	Triangular (scored)	Orange	SKF E19
Dexedrine Spansule	dextroamphetamine	5 10 15	Capsule Capsule Capsule		Brown/clear, (orange/white pellets)	SKF E12 SKF E13 (1 dot) SKF E14 (2 dots)
Didrex	benzphetamine	25 50	Tablet Tablet	Round Round (scored)	Yellow Orange	UPJOHN UPJOHN
Dilantin	diphenylhydantoin	30	Capsule		White, pink band	P-D 365
		100	Capsule		White, orange band	P-D 362
Dilantin-D-A	diphenylhydantoin	100	Capsule		White, light orange band	P-D 385
Dilantin (+ ¼ gr phenobarbital)	diphenylhydantoin phenobarbital	100 16	Capsule		White, red band	P-D 375
Dilantin (+ ½ gr phenobarbital)	diphenylhydantoin phenobarbital	100 32.5	Capsule		White, black band	P-D 531
Dolophine	methadone	5 10	Tablet Tablet	Round Round	White	Lilly™ J 64 Lilly™ J 72

Trade name	Chemical composition	Dosage (mg)	Form	Shape	Color	Special marks
Doriden	glutethimide	125	Tablet	Round	White	CIBA
		250	Tablet	Round (scored)	White	CIBA
		500	Tablet	Round (scored)	White	CIBA
		500	Capsule		Blue/white	CIBA
Ekko Jr.	diphenylhydantoin	100	Capsule		Blue/yellow	
Ekko Sr.	diphenylhydantoin	250	Capsule		Blue/yellow	
Elavil	amitriptyline	10	Tablet	Round	Blue	MSD 23
		25	Tablet	Round	Yellow	MSD 45
		50	Tablet	Round	Beige	MSD 102
Equanil	meprobamate	200	Tablet	Pentagonal (scored)	White	Wyeth™
		400	Tablet	Round (scored)	White	Wyeth™
Equanil L-A	meprobamate	400	Capsule		Red/clear (red/white pellets)	
Equanil Wyseals	meprobamate	400	Tablet	Round	Yellow	Wyeth™
Eskabarb Spansule	phenobarbital	65	Capsule		Blue/clear (blue/white/pellets)	SKF H74 (1 dot)
		97.5	Capsule		Blue/clear (blue/white pellets)	SKF H76 (2 dots)
Eskalith	lithium carbonate	300	Capsule		Grey/yellow	SKF J07
Eskaphen B	phenobarbital thiamine	16 5	Tablet	Round	Pink	SKF J20

Etrafon	perphenazine amitriptyline	2 25	Tablet	Round	Pink	Schering™ ANC
Etrafon 2-10	perphenazine amitriptyline	2 10	Tablet	Round	Yellow	Schering™ ANA
Etrafon-A	perphenazine amitriptyline	4 10	Tablet	Round	Orange	Schering™ ANB
Etrafon-forte	perphenazine amitriptyline	4 25	Tablet	Round	Red	Schering™ ANE
Eutonyl	pargyline	10 25 50	Tablet Tablet Tablet	Round Round Round	Pink Apricot Blue	Abbott™ Abbott™ Abbott™
Felsules	chloral hydrate	244 487 65	Capsule Capsule Capsule	Oval	White/blue Blue Yellow	400 FELLOWS 405 FELLOWS 410
Frenquel	azacyclonol	20 100	Tablet Tablet	Round Round	Blue White	Merrell™ Merrell™
Gemonil	metharbital	100	Tablet	Round (scored)	White	Abbott™
Haldol	haloperidol	.5 1 2 5	Tablet Tablet Tablet Tablet	Round (scored) Round (scored) Round (scored) Round	White Yellow Pink Green	MCNEIL ½ MCNEIL 1 MCNEIL 2 MCNEIL 5
Kemadrin	procyclidine	2 5	Tablet Tablet	Round Round (scored)	White White	F4B
Kesso-Bamate	meprobamate	200 400	Tablet Tablet	Round Round	White White	McKesson™

Trade name	Chemical composition	Dosage (mg)	Form	Shape	Color	Special marks
Kessodanten	diphenylhydantoin	100	Capsule		Green/white	McKesson™
Kessodrate	chloral hydrate	250	Capsule		Red	McKesson™
		500	Capsule		Red	McKesson™
Largactil	chlorpromazine	10	Tablet	Round	White	Poulenc™
		25	Tablet	Round (scored)	White	Poulenc™
		50	Tablet	Round	White	Poulenc™ cross imprint
		100	Tablet	Round (cross scored)	White	Poulenc™
Libritabs	chlordiazepoxide	5	Tablet	Round	Green	ROCHE
		10	Tablet	Round	Green	ROCHE
		25	Tablet	Round	Green	ROCHE
Librium	chlordiazepoxide	5	Capsule		Green/yellow	ROCHE 1
		10	Capsule		Green/black	ROCHE 2
		25	Capsule		Green/white	ROCHE 3
Listica	hydroxyphenamate	200	Tablet	Round	White	Armour
Lithane	lithium carbonate	300	Tablet	Round (scored)	Green	ROERIG 566
Lithonate	lithium carbonate	300	Capsule		Pink (flesh)	Rowell
Lotusate	talbutal	30	Tablet	Capsule-shaped	Yellow	W
		120	Tablet	Capsule-shaped	Purple	W
Luminal	phenobarbital	16	Tablet	Ovoid	White	Winthrop™

Brand	Generic	Strength	Form	Shape	Color	Manufacturer
		32	Tablet	Ovoid	White	Winthrop™
Majeptil	thioproperazine	1	Tablet	Round	White	Poulenc™ (diamond imprint)
		1	Tablet	Round (scored)	Orange	Poulenc™
		5	Tablet	Round (scored)	Orange	Poulenc™
		10	Tablet	Round	Orange	Poulenc™ (cross imprint)
Marplan	isocarboxazid	10	Tablet	Round (scored)	Peach	ROCHE
Mebaral	mephobarbital	32	Tablet	Round (scored)	White	Winthrop™ (3 dots)
		50	Tablet	Round	White	Winthrop™ (3 lines)
		100	Tablet	Round	White	Winthrop™ (1 dot)
		200	Tablet	Round (scored)	White	Winthrop™ (3 dots)
Mebroin	mephobarbital diphenylhydantoin	90 / 60	Tablet	Round (scored)	Orange (mottled)	Winthrop™
Medomin (discontinued 1970)	heptabarbital	200	Tablet	Round (scored)	White	Geigy
Mellaril	thioridazine	10	Tablet	Round	Chartreuse, bright	SANDOZ 78-2 10
		25	Tablet	Round	Tan	SANDOZ 78-3 25
		50	Tablet	Round	White	SANDOZ 78-4 50
		100	Tablet	Round	Chartreuse, light	SANDOZ 78-5 100
		150	Tablet	Round	Yellow	SANDOZ 78-6 150
		200	Tablet	Round	Pink	SANDOZ 78-7 200
Meprospan	meprobamate	200	Capsule		Yellow/clear (yellow/white pellets)	WALLACE 200

Trade name	Chemical composition	Dosage (mg)	Form	Shape	Color	Special marks
		400	Capsule		Blue/clear (yellow/white pellets)	WALLACE 400
Meprotab	meprobamate	400	Tablet	Round	White	
Mesantoin	mephenytoin	100	Tablet	Round (scored)	Pink	SANDOZ™ 78-52
Methadone	methadone	5	Tablet	Round	Purple (mottled)	CRW
Methedrine	methamphetamine	2.5	Tablet	Round (scored)	White	Burroughs Wellcome™
		5	Tablet	Round (scored)	White	Burroughs Wellcome™
Metrazol	pentylenetetrazol	100	Tablet	Round	White	K
Milontin	phensuximide	250	Capsule		Orange/white, red band	P-D 399
		500	Capsule		Orange, orange band	P-D 393
Miltown	meprobamate	200	Tablet	Round	White	Wallace™
		400	Tablet	Round (scored)	White	Wallace™
Mysoline	primidone	50	Tablet	Round (scored)	White	Ayerst 431
		250	Tablet	Round (scored)	White	Ayerst 430
Nardi[1]	phenelzine	15	Tablet	Round	Orange	W/C

Name	Drug	Strength (mg)	Form	Shape	Color	Code
Navane	thiothixene	1	Capsule		Yellow/Orange	571 (1 mg)
		2	Capsule		Yellow/Aqua	572 (2 mg)
		5	Capsule		Orange/white	573 (5 mg)
		10	Capsule		White/Aqua	574 (10 mg)
Nembutal	sodium pentobarbital	30	Capsule		Yellow	Abbott[TM]
		50	Capsule		Clear/yellow	Abbott[TM]
		100	Capsule		Yellow	Abbott[TM]
Nembutal Gradumet	sodium pentobarbital	100	Tablet	Round	Blue	Abbott
Niamid	nialamide	25	Tablet	Round (scored)	Violet	Pfizer 532
		100	Tablet	Round (scored)	Pink	Pfizer 533
Nioric	pentylenetetrazol	100	Tablet	Round	White	Ascher[TM] 225–260
Noctec	chloral hydrate	250	Capsule		Red	Squibb 623
		500	Capsule		Red	Squibb 626
Noludar	methyprylon	50	Tablet	Round (scored)	White	ROCHE[TM]
		200	Tablet	Round (scored)	White	ROCHE[TM]
		300	Capsule		Purple/white	ROCHE 19
Norpramin	desipramine	25	Tablet	Round	Yellow	Lakeside[TM]
		50	Tablet	Round	Green, light	Lakeside[TM]
Obedrin	methamphetamine pentobarbital	5 20	Capsule		Orange/gray	
	methamphetamine pentobarbital	5 20	Tablet	Round (scored)	Yellow	
Obedrin L-A	methamphetamine pentobarbital	12.5 50	Tablet	Round	White/pink mottled	

Trade name	Chemical composition	Dosage (mg)	Form	Shape	Color	Special marks
Obetrol	methamphetamine saccharate	2.5	Tablet	Round (scored)	Blue	OP
	methamphetamine	2.5				
	amphetamine sulfate	2.5				
	dextroamphetamine sulfate	2.5				
	methamphetamine saccharate	5	Tablet	Round (scored)	Orange	OP
	methamphetamine	5				
	amphetamine sulfate	5				
	dextroamphetamine sulfate	5				
Obotan	dextroamphetamine tannate	17.5	Tablet	Flat oblong	Olive green	
Obotan Forte	dextroamphetamine tannate	26.25	Tablet	Flat oblong	Violet gray	
Obotan-S	dextroamphetamine tannate	17.5	Tablet	Flat oblong (scored)	Orange	
	secobarbital	35				
Olbese No. 1	amobarbital	50	Tablet	Flat oblong	Blue/white (speckled)	
	methamphetamine	10				
Pacatal	mepazine	25	Tablet	Round (scored)	White	Warner-Chilcott™
Paradione	paramethadione	50	Tablet	Round (scored)	White	Warner-Chilcott™
		150	Capsule	Round	Red	
		300	Capsule	Round	Red	

Paral	paraldehyde	975	Capsule		Red	FELLOWS 730
Parest	methaqualone	200	Capsule		Turquoise/green	P-D 572
		400	Capsule		Blue/green	P-D 574
Parnate	tranylcypromine	10	Tablet	Round	Red	SKF 10, N71
Pedestal	levo-amphetamine succinate	7	Tablet	Flat oblong	Pink/blue mottled	
		21	Capsule		Clear (orange/yellow pellets)	
Peganone	ethotoin	250	Tablet	Round (scored)	White	Abbott^{TM}
		500	Tablet	Round (scored)	White	Abbott^{TM}
Penotal	phenobarbital pentobarbital					Coastal
Pentobarbital	pentobarbital	100	Capsule			Lilly^{TM} F90
PERKé ONE	dextroamphetamine	15	Capsule		Red/clear (white pellet)	
PERKé TWO	dextroamphetamine amobarbital	15 60	Capsule		Red/yellow clear	
Permitil	fluphenazine	.25	Tablet	Round	Green	WBK
		1	Tablet	Oval (scored)	Yellow	$\frac{W}{L}$ WGB
		2.5	Tablet	Oval (scored)	Orange	$\frac{W}{L}$ WDR
		5	Tablet	Oval (scored)	Purple	$\frac{W}{L}$ WFF
		10	Tablet	Oval (scored)	Rose	$\frac{W}{L}$ WFG

Trade name	Chemical composition	Dosage (mg)	Form	Shape	Color	Special marks
Permitil Chronotab	fluphenazine	1	Tablet	Round	Yellow	WKJ
Pertofrane	desipramine	25	Capsule		Pink	Geigy™ 05
		50	Capsule		Pink/maroon	Geigy™ 07
Phelantin	phenobarbital	30	Capsule		Yellow, orange band	P-D 394
	diphenylhydantoin	100				
	methamphetamine	2.5				
Phenergan	promethazine	12.5	Tablet	Round (scored)	Gray	Wyeth™
		25	Tablet	Round (scored)	White	Wyeth™
		50	Tablet	Round	Pink	Wyeth™
Phenobarbital	phenobarbital	15	Tablet	Round	White	Lilly™ J31
		30	Tablet	Round	White	Lilly™ J32
		60	Tablet	Round	White	Lilly™ J37
		100	Tablet	Round	White	Lilly™ J33
Phenurone	phenacemide	500	Tablet	Round (scored)	White	Abbott™
Placidyl	ethchlorvynol	100	Capsule	Round	Red	
		200	Capsule	Round	Red	
		500	Capsule	Capsule	Red	ABBOTT
		750	Capsule		Green	ABBOTT
Plexonal	sodium diethylbarbiturate	45	Tablet	Triangular	White	Sandoz™ 78-57
	sodium phenylethylbarbiturate	15				

	sodium isobutylallyl-barbiturate	25				
	scopolamine bromide	.08				
	dihydroergotamine methanesulfonate	.16				
Preludin	phenmetrazine	25	Tablet	Square (scored)	Pink	Geigy^{TM} 42
		75	Tablet	Round	Pink	Geigy^{TM} 62
Proketazine	carphenazine	12.5	Tablet	Round	Yellow	
		25	Tablet	Round	Orange	
		50	Tablet	Round	Rose	
Prolixin	fluphenazine	1	Tablet	Round	Pink	Squibb^{TM} 863
		2.5	Tablet	Round	Yellow	Squibb^{TM} 864
		5	Tablet	Round	Green	Squibb^{TM} 877
Providex	dextroamphetamine sulfate	15	Tablet	Round	White/blue mottled	
	amobarbital	60				
Quaalude	methaqualone	150	Tablet	Round (scored)	White	WHR
		300	Tablet	Round (scored)	White	RORER
Quadamine	dextroamphetamine sulfate	15	Capsue		Blue/clear, aqua band (red/blue pellets)	TUTAG
	amobarbital	45				
	vitamins					
Quide	piperacetazine	10	Tablet	Round	Orange	
		25	Tablet	Round	Yellow	

Trade name	Chemical composition	Dosage (mg)	Form	Shape	Color	Special marks
Repoise	butaperazine	5	Tablet	Round	Yellow	AHR
		10	Tablet	Round	Green	AHR
		25	Tablet	Round	Orange	AHR
Ritalin	methylphenidate	5	Tablet	Round	Yellow	CIBA
		10	Tablet	Round	Pale green	CIBA
		20	Tablet	Round (scored)	Peach	CIBA
Sansert	methysergide	2	Tablet	Round	Yellow	SANDOZ™ 78–58
Seconal	secobarbital	30	Capsule		Orange	Lilly™ (30 mg) F72
		50	Capsule	Round	Orange	Lilly™ (50 mg) F42
		100	Capsule	Round	Orange	Lilly™ (100 mg) F40
Serax	oxazepam	10	Capsule		Pink/white	WYETH 10
		15	Capsule		Red/white	WYETH 15
		15	Tablet	Round	Yellow	WYETH™
		30	Capsule		Maroon/white	WYETH 30
Serentil	mesoridazine	10	Tablet	Round	Rose	Sandoz 78-11
		25	Tablet	Round	Rose	Sandoz 78-12
		50	Tablet	Round	Rose	Sandoz 78-13
		100	Tablet	Round	Rose	Sandoz 78-14
Sinequan	doxepin	10	Capsule		Pink/red	Pfizer 10 534
		25	Capsule		Turquoise/pink	Pfizer 25 535
		50	Capsule		Pink/light pink	Pfizer 50 536

Softran	buclizine	25	Tablet	Round (scored)	White	Stuart
		50	Tablet	Round (scored)	Red	Stuart
Solacen	tybamate	250	Capsule	Ovoid	Yellow	
		350	Capsule	Ovoid	Yellow	
Somnafac	methaqualone	200	Capsule		Two-tone blue	
		400	Capsule		Dark blue	
Somnos	chloral hydrate	32.5	Capsule		Red	Merck 641
Sopor	methaqualone	75	Tablet	Round (scored)	Green	AS
		150	Tablet	Round (scored)	Yellow	AS
		300	Tablet	Round (scored)	Orange	AS
Sparine	promazine	10	Tablet	Round	Green	
		25	Tablet	Round	Yellow	
		50	Tablet	Round	Orange	
		100	Tablet	Round	Pink	
		200	Tablet	Round	Red	
Stelazine	trifluoperazine	1	Tablet	Round	Blue	SKF 1 SO3
		2	Tablet	Round	Blue	SKF 2 SO4
		5	Tablet	Round	Blue	SKF 5 SO6
		10	Tablet	Round	Blue	SKF 10 SO7
Stental	phenobarbital	48.6	Tablet	Round	Pink	AHR
Suavitil	benactyzine	1	Tablet	Round (scored)	White	Merck™
Surmontil	trimipramine	25	Tablet	Round (scored)	Red	Poulenc™
		100	Tablet	Round (scored)	Red	Poulenc™

Trade name	Chemical composition	Dosage (mg)	Form	Shape	Color	Special marks
Taractan	chlorprothixene	10	Tablet	Round	Red	ROCHE 10
		25	Tablet	Round	Red	ROCHE 25
		50	Tablet	Round	Red	ROCHE 50
		100	Tablet	Round	Red	ROCHE 100
Tegretol	carbamazepine	200	Tablet	Round (scored)	White	GEIGY™ 67
Thorazine	chlorpromazine	10	Tablet	Round	Orange	SKF 10 T73
		25	Tablet	Round	Orange	SKF 25 T74
		50	Tablet	Round	Orange	SKF 50 T76
		100	Tablet	Round	Orange	SKF 100 T77
		200	Tablet	Round	Orange	SKF 200 T79
Thorazine Spansules	chlorpromazine	30	Capsule		Orange/clear, (orange/white pellets)	SKF T63 (1 dot)
		75	Capsule			SKF T64 (2 dots)
		150	Capsule			SKF T66 (3 dots)
		200	Capsule			SKF T67 (4 dots)
		300	Capsule			SKF T69 (5 dots)
Tindal	acetophenazine	20	Tablet	Round	Rose	Schering™ BBA
Tofranil	imipramine	10	Tablet	Triangular	Coral	Geigy™ 21
		25	Tablet	Round	Coral	Geigy™ 11
		50	Tablet	Round	Coral	Geigy™ 74
Toin Unicelles	diphenylhydantoin	125	Capsule		Gray/clear, pink band, (pink & white pellets)	Reid-Provident™
		250	Capsule		White/clear, black band, (gray pellets)	Reid-Provident™

Name	Ingredients	Strength	Form	Shape	Color	Manufacturer
Trancopal	chlormethazanone	100	Tablet	Capsule-shaped (scored)	Orange	Winthrop™
		200	Tablet	Capsule-shaped (scored)	Green	Winthrop™
Triavil	perphenazine amitriptyline	2 / 10	Tablet	Triangular	Blue	MSD 914
	perphenazine amitriptyline	2 / 25	Tablet	Triangular	Orange	MSD 921
	perphenazine amitriptyline	4 / 10	Tablet	Triangular	Salmon	MSD 934
	perphenazine amitriptyline	4 / 25	Tablet	Triangular	Yellow	MSD 946
Tridione	trimethadione	150	Tablet	Square	White	Abbott™
		300	Capsule		White	Abbott™
Trilafon	perphenazine	2	Tablet	Round	White	Schering™ (black) ADH
		4	Tablet	Round	White	Schering™ (blue) ADK
		8	Tablet	Round	White	Schering™ (green) ADJ
		16	Tablet	Round	White	Schering™ (red) ADM
Trilafon Repetabs	perphenazine	8	Tablet	Round	White	Schering™ (black) ADX
Tuinal	secobarbital amobarbital	25 / 25	Capsule		Orange/blue	Lilly™ F64
	secobarbital amobarbital	50 / 50	Capsule		Orange/blue	Lilly™ F65

Trade name	Chemical composition	Dosage (mg)	Form	Shape	Color	Special marks
	secobarbital amobarbital	100 100	Capsule		Orange/blue	Lilly™ F66
Tybatran	tybamate	125 250 350	Capsule		Green	AHR 125 AHR 250 AHR 350
Ultran	phenaglycodol	200	Tablet	Capsule-shaped (scored)	Green	Lilly™ T97
		300	Capsule			Lilly™ H01
Valium	diazepam	2	Tablet	Round (scored)	White	ROCHE
		5	Tablet	Round (scored)	Yellow	ROCHE 5
		10	Tablet	Round (scored)	Blue	ROCHE 6
Valmid	ethinamate	500	Tablet	Round (scored)	Peach	Lilly™ J12
Vesprin	trifluromazine	10 25 50	Tablet Tablet Tablet	Round Round Round	Light violet Yellow Green	Squibb™ 921 Squibb™ 922 Squibb™ 923
Vistaril	hydroxyzine	25 50 100	Capsule Capsule Capsule		Two-tone green Green/white Green/gray	Pfizer 541 Pfizer 542 Pfizer 543
Vivactil	protriptyline	5 10	Tablet Tablet	Oval Oval	Orange Yellow	MSD 26 MSD 47
Zarontin	ethosuximide	250	Capsule		Orange	P-D 237

IDENTIFICATION OF TABLETS BY COLOR, SHAPE, SPECIAL MARKS, TRADE NAME, CHEMICAL COMPOSITION, AND DRUG TYPE

Color	Shape	Special marks[a]	Trade name	Chemical composition	Dosage (mg)	Drug type[c]
Blue						
Blue	Round	Abbott[TM][b] (geometric "a")	Eutonyl	pargyline	50	Antidepressant
			Nembutal	pentobarbital	100	Sedative
Blue	Round	MSD 23	Elavil	amitriptyline	10	Antidepressant
Blue	Round	Merrell[TM]	Frenquel	azacyclonol	20	Antianxiety
Blue	Round (scored)	OP	Obetrol-10	methamphetamine saccharate	2.5	—[c]
				methamphetamine	2.5	
				amphetamine sulfate	2.5	
				dextroamphetamine sulfate	2.5	
Blue	Round	SKF 1 SO3	Stelazine	trifluoperazine	1	Antipsychotic
		SKF 2 SO4	Stelazine	trifluoperazine	2	Antipsychotic
		SKF 5 SO6	Stelazine	trifluoperazine	5	Antipsychotic
		SKF 10 SO7	Stelazine	trifluoperazine	10	Antipsychotic
Blue	Round (scored)	TUTAG	Cydril	levamphetamine succinate	7	Stimulant
Blue	Round (scored)	ROCHE 6	Valium	diazepam	10	Antianxiety
Blue	Triangular	MSD 914	Triavil	perphenazine	2	
				amitriptyline	10	
Blue/ white	Round		Adipex	methamphetamine	10	
				amobarbital	50	

Blue/ white, mottled	Round		Providex	dextroamphetamine amobarbital	15 60	
Blue/ white, mottled	Flat oblong		Olbese No. 1	methamphetamine amobarbital	10 50	
Blue/ pink, mottled	Flat oblong		Pedestal	levamphetamine	7	Stimulant
Blue/ orange	Round	Abbott™	Desbutal 10	methamphetamine pentobarbital	10 60	
Blue/ yellow	Round	Abbott™	Desbutal 15	methamphetamine pentobarbital	15 90	
Brown						
Brown (beige)	Round	MSD 102	Elavil	amitriptyline	50	Antidepressant
Brown (tan)	Round	25 78–3 Sandoz	Mellaril	thioridazine	25	Antipsychotic
Gray						
Gray	Round (scored)	Wyeth™	Phenergan	promethazine	12.5	Antipsychotic

[a]Tablets may or may not have code numbers or letters, according to date of manufacture. All drug companies will eventually manufacture all medications with identification code.

[b]TM stands for trademark which may be company name or symbol.

[c]Drug type not indicated for combination drugs.

Color	Shape	Special marks[a]	Trade name	Chemical composition	Dosage (mg)	Drug type[c]
Green						
Green	Round		Sparine	promazine	10	Antipsychotic
Green	Round	Palmedico TM	Amphaplex 20	methamphetamine saccharate	5	
				methamphetamine hydrochloride		
				amphetamine	5	
				dextroamphetamine	5	
Green	Round	561	Atarax	hydroxyzine	25	Antianxiety
					5	
Green	Round	ROCHE	Libritabs	chlordiazepoxide	10	Antianxiety
					25	
Green (chartreuse)	Round	Sandoz 10 78-2	Mellaril	thioridazine	10	Antipsychotic
	Round	Sandoz 100 78-5			100	
Green	Round	Lakeside TM	Norpramin	desipramine	50	Antidepressant
Green	Round	WBK	Permitil	fluphenazine	0.25	Antianxiety
Green	Round	Squibb TM 877	Prolixin	fluphenazine	5	Antipsychotic
Green	Round	AHR	Repoise	butaperazine	10	Antipsychotic
Green	Round	CIBA	Ritalin	methylphenidate	10	Stimulant
Green	Round	Squibb TM 923	Vesprin	triflupromazine	50	Antipsychotic
Green	Round (scored)	McNeil	Butisol	butabarbital	30	Sedative

Color	Shape	Code	Trade name	Generic name	Strength	Category
Green	Round (scored)	McNeil 5	Haldol	haloperidol	5	Antipsychotic
Green	Round (scored)	Roerig 566	Lithane	lithium carbonate	300	Antimanic
Green	Round (scored)	A / S	Sopor	methaqualone	75	Hypnotic
Green (olive)	Capsule-shaped	Lilly™ T40	Obotan	dextroamphetamine	17.5	Stimulant
Green (light)	Flat, oblong		Amytal	amobarbital	15	Sedative
Green	Triangular (scored)	SKF D93	Dexamyl	dextroamphetamine / amobarbital	5 / 32	
Green	Capsule-shaped (scored)	Winthrop™	Trancopal	chlormethazanone	200	Antianxiety
Green	Capsule-shaped (scored)	Lilly™ T97	Ultran	phenaglycodol	200	Antianxiety

Orange

Color	Shape	Code	Trade name	Generic name	Strength	Category
Orange	Round		Proketazine / Quide / Sparine	carphenazine / piperacetazine / promazine	25 / 10 / 50	Antipsychotic / Antipsychotic / Antipsychotic
Orange	Round	560	Atarax	hydroxyzine	10	Antianxiety
Orange	Round	Abbott™	Desoxyn	methamphetamine	10	Stimulant
Orange	Round	Schering™ ANB	Etrafon-A	perphenazine / amitriptyline	4 / 10	
Orange (apricot)	Round	Abbott™	Eutonyl	pargyline	25	Antidepressant

Color	Shape	Special marks[a]	Trade name	Chemical composition	Dosage (mg)	Drug type[c]
Orange	Round	Knoll[TM]	Metrazol Vita-M	pentylenetetrazol vitamins	100	
Orange	Round	Poulenc[TM] (cross imprint)	Majeptil	thioproperazine	10	Antipsychotic
Orange	Round	W/C	Nardil	phenelzine	15	Antidepressant
Orange	Round	AHR	Repoise	butaperazine	25	Antipsychotic
Orange	Round	SKF 10 T73	Thorazine	chlorpromazine	10	Antipsychotic
		SKF 25 T74	Thorazine	chlorpromazine	25	
		SKF 50 T76	Thorazine	chlorpromazine	50	
		SKF 100 T77	Thorazine	chlorpromazine	100	
		SKF 200 T79	Thorazine	chorpromazine	200	
Orange (coral)	Round	Geigy[TM] 11	Tofranil	imipramine	25	Antidepressant
		Geigy[TM] 74	Tofranil	imipramine	50	Antidepressant
Orange	Round (scored)	McNeil[TM]	Butisol Sodium	Sodium butabarbital	50	Sedative
Orange	Round (scored)	Upjohn[TM]	Didrex	benzphetamine	50	Stimulant
Orange	Round (scored)	Poulenc[TM]	Majeptil	thioproperazine	1	Antipsychotic
				thioproperazine	5	Antipsychatic
Orange (peach)	Round (scored)	Roche[TM]	Marplan	isocarboxazid	10	Antidepressant
Orange	Round (scored)	OP	Obetrol-20	methamphetamine saccharate	5	
				methamphetamine hydrochloride	5	

Color	Shape	Code	Trade Name	Ingredient	mg	Category
				amphetamine sulfate	5	Stimulant
				dextroamphetamine sulfate	5	
Orange (peach)	Round (scored)	CIBA	Ritalin	methylphenidate	20	Stimulant
Orange	Round (scored)	A S	Sopor	methaqualone	300	Hypnotic
Orange (peach)	Round (scored)	Lilly J12	Valmid	ethinamate	500	Hypnotic
Orange	Oval	MSD 26	Vivactil	protriptyline	5	Antidepressant
Orange	Oval (scored)	$\frac{W}{L}$ WDR	Permitil	fluphenazine	2.5	Antipsychotic
Orange	Flat oblong (scored)	Lilly^{TM} T37	Amytal	amobarbital	50	Sedative
Orange	Capsule-shaped (scored)	—	Obotan-S	dextroamphetamine tannate	17.5	
				secobarbital	35	
Orange	Capsule-shaped (scored)	Winthrop^{TM}	Trancopal	chlormethazanone	100	Antianxiety
Orange (coral)	Triangular	Geigy^{TM} 21	Tofranil	imipramine	10	Antidepressant
Orange	Triangular	MSD 921	Triavil	perphenazine	2	
				amitriptyline	25	
Orange	Triangular (scored)	SKF E19	Dexedrine	dextroamphetamine	5	Stimulant
Orange (mottled)	Round (scored)	Winthrop^{TM}	Mebroin	mephobarbital	90	Anticonvulsant
				diphenylhydantoin	60	

Color	Shape	Special marks[a]	Trade name	Chemical composition	Dosage (mg)	Drug type[c]
Orange/blue	Round	Abbott TM	Desbutal 10 Gradumet	methamphetamine sodium pentobarbital	10 60	
Pink						
Pink	Round		Bamadex	dextroamphetamine meprobamate	5 400	
Pink	Round	Abbott TM	Sparine	promazine	100	Antipsychotic
Pink	Round	Abbott TM	Eutonyl	pargyline	10	Antidepressant
Pink	Round	Wallace TM	Harmonyl	deserpidine	0.25	Antipsychotic
Pink	Round		Deprol	meprobamate benactyzine	400 1	
Pink	Round	SKF J20	Eskaphen B	phenobarbital thiamine	16 5	
Pink	Round	Schering TM ANC	Etrafon	perphenazine amitryptyline	2 25	
Pink	Round	Sandoz TM 200 78-7	Mellaril	thioridazine	200	Antipsychotic
Pink	Round	Wyeth TM	Phenergan	promethazine	50	Antipsychotic
Pink	Round	Geigy TM 62	Preludin Endurets	phenmetrazine	75	Stimulant
Pink	Round	Squibb TM 863	Prolixin	fluphenazine	1	Antipsychotic
Pink	Round	AHR	Stental	phenobarbital	48.6	Sedative
Pink	Round (scored)	Palmedico TM	Amphaplex 10	methamphetamine saccharate	2.5	

Color	Shape	Code	Brand	Ingredient	Amount	Class
				methamphetamine hydrochloride amphetamine sulfate dextroamphetamine sulfate	2.5 2.5 2.5	
Pink	Round (scored)	McNeil™	Butisol Sodium	sodium butabarbital	100	Sedative
Pink	Round (scored)	Riker™	Deaner	deanol	100	Stimulant
Pink	Round (scored)	McNeil™	Haldol	haloperidol	2	Antipsychotic
Pink	Round (scored)	Sandoz™ 78-52	Mesantoin	mephenytoin	100	Anticonvulsant
Pink	Round (scored)	Pfizer™ 533	Niamid	nialamide	100	Antidepressant
Pink	Flat oblong (scored)	Lilly™ T32	Amytal	amobarbital	100	Sedative
Pink	Square (scored)	Geigy™ 42	Preludin	phenmetrazine	25	Stimulant
Pink (salmon)	Triangular (scored)	MSD 934	Triavil	perphenazine amitriptyline	4 10	
Pink	Triangular (scored)	A91	Benzedrine	amphetamine	5	Stimulant
Pink	Triangular (scored)	A92	Benzedrine	amphetamine	10	Stimulant
Pink (mottled)	Oval	MJ	Beta-Chlor	chloral betaine	870	Sedative

Color	Shape	Special marks[a]	Trade name	Chemical composition	Dosage (mg)	Drug type[c]
Pink/blue (mottled)	Flat oblong		Pedestal	levamphetamine	7	Stimulant
Pink/white (mottled)	Round		Obedrin-LA	methamphetamine pentobarbital vitamins	12.5 50	
Purple						
Purple (light violet)	Round	Squibb 921	Vesprin	triflupromazine	10	Antipsychotic
Purple (lavender)	Round (scored)	McNeil	Butisol	sodium butabarbital	15	Sedative
Purple (violet)	Round (scored)	Pfizer 532	Niamid	nialamide	25	Antidepressant
Purple	Oval (scored)	$\frac{W}{L}$ WFF	Permitil	fluphenazine	5	Antipsychotic
Purple (violet gray)	Flat oblong		Obotan-Forte	dextroamphetamine tannate	26.25	Stimulant
Purple (mottled)	Round	CRW	Methadone	methadone	5	Heroin substitute
Red						
Red (rose)	Round		Proketazine	carphenazine	50	Antipsychotic
Red	Round		Sparine	promazine	200	Antipsychotic

Color	Shape	Code	Brand	Generic	Strength	Category
Red	Round	563	Atarax	hydroxyzine	100	Antianxiety
Red	Round	Searle	Dartal	thiopropazate	2	Antipsychotic
				thiopropazate	5	Antipsychotic
				thiopropazate	10	Antipsychotic
Red	Round	Schering™ ANE	Etrafon-Forte	perphenazine	4	Antidepressant
				amitriptyline	25	
Red	Round	SKF 10 N71	Parnate	tranylcypromine	10	Antidepressant
Red (rose)	Round	Sandoz™ 78–11	Serentil	mesoridazine	10	Antipsychotic
		Sandoz™ 78–12	Serentil	mesoridazine	25	Antipsychotic
		Sandoz™ 78–13	Serentil	mesoridazine	50	Antipsychotic
		Sandoz™ 78–14	Serentil	mesoridazine	100	Antipsychotic
Red	Round	ROCHE 10	Taractan	chlorprothixene	10	Antipsychotic
		ROCHE 25	Taractan	chlorprothixene	25	Antipsychotic
		ROCHE 50	Taractan	chlorprothixene	50	Antipsychotic
		ROCHE 100	Taractan	chlorprothixene	100	Antipsychotic
Red (rose)	Round	Schering™ BBA	Tindal	acetophenazine	20	Antipsychotic
Red	Round (scored)	Stuart	Softran	buclizine	50	Antianxiety
Red	Round (scored)	Poulenc™	Surmontil	trimipramine	25	Antidepressant
					100	
Red (rose)	Oval (scored)	W/L WFG	Permitil	fluphenazine	10	Antipsychotic

White

Color	Shape	Code	Brand	Generic	Strength	Category
White	Round	Abbott™	Desoxyn	methamphetamine	2.5	Stimulant
					5	

Color	Shape	Special marks[a]	Trade name	Chemical composition	Dosage (mg)	Drug type[c]
White	Round		Kemadrin	procyclidine	5	Antiparkinson
White	Round	Ascher[TM] 225–260	Nioric	pentylenetetrazol	100	Stimulant
White	Round	CIBA	Doriden	glutethimide	125	Hypnotic
White	Round	F 4 B	Kemadrin	procyclidine	2	Antiparkinson
White	Round	Knoll[TM]	Bromural	bromisovalum	324	Antianxiety
White	Round	K	Metrazol	pentylenetetrazol	100	Stimulant
White	Round	Lilly[TM] J64	Dolophine	methadone	5	Heroin
		Lilly[TM] J72	Dolophine	methadone	10	substitute
White	Round	Lilly J31	Phenobarbital	phenobarbital	15	Sedative
		Lilly J32	Phenobarbital	phenobarbital	30	Sedative
		Lilly J33	Phenobarbital	phenobarbital	100	Sedative
		Lilly J37	Phenobarbital	phenobarbital	60	Sedative
White	Round	MK in oval outline	Kesso-bamate	meprobamate	200	Antianxiety
			Kesso-bamate	meprobamate	400	Antianxiety
White	Round	McNeil[TM] in lavender	Butisol	sodium butabarbital	30	Sedative
		McNeil[TM] in green	Butisol	sodium butabarbital	60	Sedative
White	Round (scored)	McNeil[TM] ½	Haldol	haloperidol	0.5	Antipsychotic
White	Round	Merrel[TM]	Frenquel	azacyclonol	100	Antianxiety
White	Round	Poulenc[TM] (diamond imprint)	Majeptil	thioproperazine	1	Antipsychotic

Color	Shape	Markings	Brand	Generic	mg	Category
White	Round	Sandoz 50 78-4	Mellaril	thioridazine	50	Antipsychotic
White	Round	Schering^TM (in black) ADH	Trilafon	perphenazine	2	Antipsychotic
		Schering (in blue) ADK	Trilafon	perphenazine	4	Antipsychotic
		Schering^TM (in green) ADJ	Trilafon	perphenazine	8	Antipsychotic
White	Round	Schering^TM	Trilafon	perphenazine	16	Antipsychotic
		Schering^TM (in black) ADX	Trilafon Repetabs	perphenazine	8	Antipsychotic
White	Round	Searle	Dartal	thiopropazate	5	Antipsychotic
White	Round	Wallace ^TM	Miltown	meprobamate	200	Antianxiety
				meprobamate	400	Antianxiety
White	Round	3 lines Winthrop^TM	Mebaral	mephobarbital	50	Sedative
		1 dot Winthrop^TM	Mebaral	mephobarbital	100	Sedative
White	Round (scored)	Artane	Artane	trihexyphenidyl	2	Antiparkinson
				trihexyphenidyl	5	Antiparkinson
White	Round (scored)	Abbott^TM	Phenurone	phenacemide	500	Anticonvulsant
White	Round (scored)	Abbott^TM	Peganone	ethotoin	250	Anticonvulsant
		Abbott^TM	Peganone	ethotoin	500	Anticonvulsant
		Abbott^TM	Gemonil	metharbital	100	Sedative
White	Round (scored)	Ayerst^TM 430	Mysoline	primidone	250	Anticonvulsant
White	Round (scored)	Ayerst^TM 431	Mysoline	primidone	50	Anticonvulsant
White	Round (scored)	Ayerst^TM 809	Antabuse	disulfiram	250	Alcohol antagonist
		Ayerst^TM 810	Antabuse	disulfiram	500	antagonist

Color	Shape	Special marks[a]	Trade name	Chemical composition	Dosage (mg)	Drug type[c]
White	Round (scored)	Burroughs-Wellcome[TM]	Methedrine	methamphetamine methamphetamine	2.5 5	Stimulant Stimulant
White	Round (scored)	CIBA	Doriden Doriden	glutethimide glutethimide	250 500	Hypnotic Hypnotic
White	Round (scored)	Geigy[TM]	Medomin	heptabarbital	200	Sedative
	Round (scored)	Geigy[TM] 67	Tegretol	carbamazepine	200	Indicated for tic douloureux
White	Round (scored)	Knoll[TM]	Akineton	biperiden	2	Antiparkinson
White	Round (scored)	Merck[TM]	Suavitil	benactyzine	1	Antianxiety
White	Round (scored)	MSD 21	Cogentin	benztropine mesylate	0.5	Antiparkinson
White	Round (cross-scored)	MSD 60	Cogentin	benztropine mesylate	2	Antiparkinson
White	Round (scored)	RIKER	Deaner	deanol	25	Stimulant
White	Round (scored)	ROCHE[TM]	Noludar	methyprylon methyprylon	50 200	Hypnotic Hypnotic
White	Round (scored)	RORER	Quaalude	methaqualone	300	Hypnotic
White	Round (scored)	Roche	Valium	diazepam	2	Antianxiety

Color	Shape	Manufacturer/Marking	Trade name	Generic name	Strength	Category
White	Round (scored)	Stuart	Softran	buclizine	25	Antianxiety
White	Round (scored)	Warner-Chilcott™	Pacatal	mepazine	25	Antipsychotic
				mepazine	50	Antipsychotic
White	Round (scored)	WHR	Quaalude	methaqualone	150	Hypnotic
White	Round (scored)	Wallace™ (W inside hexagon)	Miltown	meprobamate	400	Antianxiety
White	Round (scored)	3 dots Winthrop™	Mebaral	mephobarbital	32	Sedative
White	Round (scored)	3 big dots Winthrop™	Mebaral	mephobarbital	200	Sedative
White	Round (scored)	Wyeth™ (script W inside square)	Equanil / Phenergan	meprobamate	400	Antianxiety
				promethazine	25	Antipsychotic
White	Ovoid	Winthrop™	Luminal	phenobarbital	16	Sedative
				phenobarbital	32	Sedative
White	Oval (scored)	MSD 635	Cogentin	benztropine mesylate	1	Antiparkinson
White	Pentagonal (scored tablet) (5 unequal sides)	W	Equanil	meprobamate	200	Antianxiety
White	Square	Abbott™	Tridione Dulcet	trimethadone	150	Anticonvulsant
White	Triangular	Sandoz™ 78–57	Plexonal	diethylbarbiturate	45	
				phenylethylbarbiturate	15	

Color	Shape	Special marks[a]	Trade name	Chemical composition	Dosage (mg)	Drug type[c]
				isobutylallylbarbiturate	25	
				scopalomine	.08	
				dihydroergotomine	.16	
White/blue	Round		Adipex	methamphetamine	10	
				amobarbital	50	
White/blue (mottled)	Round		Providex	dextroamphetamine	15	
				amobarbital	60	
White/blue (mottled)	Flat oblong		Olbese	methamphetamine	10	
				amobarbital	50	
White/pink (mottled)	Round		Obedrin-LA	methamphetamine	12.5	
				pentobarbital	50	
				vitamins		

Yellow

Color	Shape	Special marks[a]	Trade name	Chemical composition	Dosage (mg)	Drug type[c]
Yellow	Round		Proketazine	carphenazine	12.5	Antipsychotic
			Quide	piperacetazine	25	Antipsychotic
			Sparine	promazine	25	Antipsychotic
Yellow	Round	Abbott™	Desoxyn	methamphetamine	15	Stimulant
		Abbott™	Harmonyl	deserpidine	0.1	Antipsychotic
Yellow	Round	AHR	Repoise	butaperazine	5	Antipsychotic
Yellow	Round	CIBA	Ritalin	methylphenidate	5	Stimulant
Yellow	Round	Lakeside™	Norpramin	desipramine	25	Antidepressant
Yellow	Round	MSD 45	Elavil	amitriptyline	25	Antidepressant
Yellow	Round	Sandoz™ 150 78-6	Mellaril	thioridazine	150	Antipsychotic

Color	Shape	Code	Trade Name	Drug	Dosage	Category
Yellow	Round	Sandoz™ 78–58	Sansert	methysergide	2	Experimental
Yellow	Round	Schering™ ANA	Etrafon	perphenazine amitriptyline	2 10	
Yellow	Round (scored)	A/S	Sopor	methaqualone	150	Hypnotic
Yellow	Round	SKF 5 C66 SKF 10 C67 SKF 25 C69	Compazine Compazine Compazine	prochlorperazine prochlorperazine prochlorperazine	5 10 25	Antipsychotic Antipsychotic Antipsychotic
Yellow	Round	Squibb™ 864	Prolixin	fluphenazine	2.5	Antipsychotic
Yellow	Round	Squibb™ 922	Vesprin	triflupromazine	25	Antipsychotic
Yellow	Round	UPJOHN	Didrex	benzphetamine	25	Stimulant
Yellow	Round	WKJ	Permitil Chronostat	fluphenazine	1	Antipsychotic
Yellow	Round	Wyeth	Equanil Wyseals	meprobamate	400	Antianxiety
Yellow	Round	Wyeth	Serax	oxazepam	15	Antianxiety
Yellow	Round	562	Atarax	hydroxyzine	50	Antianxiety
Yellow	Round (scored)	Obedrin	methamphetamine pentobarbital vitamins	5 20		
Yellow	Round (scored)	MCNEIL 1	Haldol	haloperidol	1	Antipsychotic
Yellow	Round (scored)	ROCHE 5	Valium	diazepam	5	Antianxiety
Yellow	Capsule-shaped	W	Lotusate	talbutal	30	Sedative
Yellow	Flat oblong (scored)	Lilly™ T56	Amytal	amobarbital	30	Sedative

Color	Shape	Special marks[a]	Trade name	Chemical composition	Dosage (mg)	Drug type[c]
Yellow	Oval	MSD 47	Vivactil	protriptyline	10	Antidepressant
Yellow	Oval (scored)	$\dfrac{W}{L}$ WGB	Permitil	fluphenazine	1	Antipsychotic
Yellow	Triangular	MSD 946	Triavil	perhenazine amitriptyline	4 25	
Yellow/ blue	Round	Abbott™	Desbutal 15 Gradumet	methamphetamine pentobarbital	15 90	

IDENTIFICATION OF CAPSULES BY COLOR, SHAPE, SPECIAL MARKS, TRADE NAME, CHEMICAL COMPOSITION, AND DRUG TYPE

Color	Shape/form	Special marks[a]	Trade name	Chemical composition	Dosage (mg)	Drug type[c]
Black						
Black	Capsule	Strasenburgh[TMb] 18–875	Biphetamine 20	dextroamphetamine amphetamine	10 10	Stimulant
Black/clear (yellow/ white pellets)	Capsule	SKF C44 (1 dot) SKF C46 (2 dots) SKF C47 (3 dots) SKF C49 (4 dots)	Compazine Spansule	prochlorperazine prochlorperazine prochlorperazine prochlorperazine	10 15 30 75	Antipsychotic Antipsychotic Antipsychotic Antipsychotic
Black/green	Capsule	ROCHE 2	Librium	chlordiazepoxide	10	Antianxiety
		Strasenburgh[TM] 18-899	Biphetamine-T 12½	dextroamphetamine amphetamine methaqualone	6.25 6.25 40	—[c]
Black/red	Capsule	Strasenburgh[TM] 18-898	Biphetamine-T 20	methaqualone dextroamphetamine amphetamine	40 10 10	Stimulant
Black/white	Capsule	Strasenburgh[TM] 18-878	Biphetamine 12½	dextroamphetamine amphetamine	6.25 6.25	Stimulant
Blue						
Blue	Ovoid Cap	Lederle[TM]	Artane Sequel	trihexyphenidyl	5	Antiparkinson
Blue	Capsule	Lilly[TM] F23 Lilly[TM] F33 FELLOWS 405	Amytal Amytal Felsules	amobarbital amobarbital chloral hydrate	65 200 487	Sedative Sedative Sedative
Blue, dark	Capsule		Somnafac Fourte	methaqualone	400	Hypnotic

Color	Type	Code	Trade name	Generic	mg	Category
Blue, two tone	Capsule		Somnafac	methaqualone	200	Hypnotic
Blue/clear, aqua band (red/blue pellets)	Capsule	TUTAG	Quadamine	dextroamphetamine amobarbital vitamins	15 45	
Blue/clear, blue/white pellets	Capsule	SKF H74 (1 dot)	Eskabarb Spansule phenobarbital	phenobarbital	65	Sedative
		SKF H76 (2 dots)		phenobarbital	97.5	
Blue/clear, (yellow & white pellets)	Capsule	WALLACE 400	Meprospan	meprobamate	400	Antianxiety
Blue (turquoise)/green	Capsule	P-D 572	Parest 200	methaqualone	200	Hypnotic
Blue/green	Capsule	P-D 574	Parest 400	methaqualone	400	Hypnotic
Blue/orange	Capsule	Lilly^{TM} F64	Tuinal	secobarbital amobarbital	25 25	
		Lilly^{TM} F65	Tuinal	secobarbital amobarbital	50 50	Hypnotic
		Lilly^{TM} F66	Tuinal	secobarbital amobarbital	100 100	Hypnotic
Blue (turquoise)/pink	Capsule	Pfizer 25 535	Sinequan	doxepin	25	Antidepressant

[a]Capsule may or may not have code numbers or letters, according to date of manufacture. All drug companies will eventually manufacture all medications with identification code.

[b]TM stands for trademark which may be drug company name or symbol.

[c]Combination drugs not cited by type.

Color	Shape/form	Special marks[a]	Trade name	Chemical composition	Dosage (mg)	Drug type[c]
Blue/white	Capsule		Adipex	methamphetamine amobarbital	10 50	
Blue/white	Capsule	CIBA	Doriden	glutethimide	500	Hypnotic
Blue/white	Oval Cap	400	Felsules	chloral hydrate	244	Sedative
Blue (aqua)/white	Capsule	574 10mg	Navane	thiothixene	10	Antipsychotic
Blue (aqua)/yellow	Capsule	572 2mg	Navane	thiothixene	2	Antipsychotic
Blue/yellow	Capsule		Ekko Sr. Ekko Jr.	diphenylhydantoin diphenylhydantoin	250 100	Anticonvulsant
Brown						
Brown/clear (orange/white pellets)	Capsule	SKF E12 SKF E13 (1 dot) SKF E14 (2 dots)	Dexedrine Dexedrine Dexedrine	dextroamphetamine dextroamphetamine dextroamphetamine	5 10 15	Stimulant Stimulant Stimulant
Brown/yellow. clear (orange/yellow pellets)	Capsule	Fellows-Testagar™ 050	Amodex	dextroamphetamine amobarbital	15 60	
Clear						
Clear (orange yellow pellets)	Capsule		Pedestal	levoamphetamine	21	Stimulant
Clear/black (yellow/white pellets)	Capsule	SKF C44 (1 dot) SKF C46 (2 dots) SKF C47 (3 dots)	Compazine Compazine Compazine	prochlorperazine prochlorperazine prochlorperazine	10 15 30	Antipsychotic Antipsychotic Antipsychotic

Clear/blue (blue/white pellets)	Capsule	SKFC49 (4 dots)	Compazine	prochlorperazine	75	Sedative
		SKF H74 (1 dot)	Eskabarb	phenobarbital	65	Sedative
		SKF H76 (2 dots)	Eskabarb	phenobarbital	97.5	
Clear/blue (yellow/white pellets)	Capsule	WALLACE 400	Meprospan 400	meprobamate	400	Antianxiety
Clear/blue aqua band (red/blue pellets)	Capsule	TUTAG	Quadamine	dextroamphetamine	15	
				amobarbital	45	
				vitamins		
Clear/brown (orange/white pellets)	Capsule	SKF E12	Dexedrine	dextroamphetamine	5	Stimulant
		SKF E13 (1 dot)	Dexedrine	dextroamphetamine	10	Stimulant
		SKF E14 (2 dots)	Dexedrine	dextroamphetamine	15	Stimulant
Clear/purple (pink/white pellets)	Capsule	SKF A90	Benzedrine	amphetamine	15	Stimulant
Clear/red (red/white pellets)	Capsule		Equanil LA	meprobamate	400	Antianxiety
Clear/red (white pellets)	Capsule		PERKé ONE	dextroamphetamine	15	Stimulant
Clear/white, black band (gray pellets)	Capsule	Reid-Provident™	Toin Unicelles	diphenylhydantoin	250	Anticonvulsant
Clear/yellow	Capsule	Abbott™	Nembutal	pentobarbital	50	Sedative
Clear/yellow (yellow/white pellets)	Capsule	WALLACE 200	Meprospan	meprobamate	200	Antianxiety

Color	Shape/form	Special marks[a]	Trade name	Chemical composition	Dosage (mg)	Drug type[c]
Clear/gray, pink band (pink/white pellets)	Capsule	Reid-Provident	Toin Unicelles	diphenylhydantoin	125	Anticonvulsant
Clear/green (green/white pellets)	Capsule	SKF D91 (1 dot)	Dexamyl	dextroamphetamine amobarbital	10 65	
		SKF D92 (2 dots)	Dexamyl	dextroamphetamine amobarbital	15 97	
Clear/green, dark green band (yellow/green pellets)	Capsule	TUTAG	Cydril	levamphetamine	21	Stimulant
Clear/orange (orange/white pellets)	Capsule	SKF T63 (1 dot) SKF T64 (2 dots) SKF T66 (3 dots) SKF T67 (4 dots) SKF T69 (5 dots)	Thorazine Thorazine Thorazine Thorazine Thorazine	chlorpromazine chlorpromazine chlorpromazine chlorpromazine chlorpromazine	30 75 150 200 300	Antipsychotic Antipsychotic Antipsychotic Antipsychotic Antipsychotic

Gray

Color	Shape/form	Special marks[a]	Trade name	Chemical composition	Dosage (mg)	Drug type[c]
Gray/clear pink band (pink & white pellets)	Capsule	Reid-Provident™	Toin Unicelles	diphenylhydantoin	125	Anticonvulsant
Gray/green	Capsule	Pfizer 543	Vistaril	hydroxyzine	100	Antianxiety

Color	Type	Code	Trade name	Drug	Amount	Class
Gray/orange	Capsule		Obedrin	methamphetamine	5 / 20	
Gray/yellow	Capsule	SKF J07	Eskalith	lithium carbonate	300	Antimanic

Green

Color	Type	Code	Trade name	Drug	Amount	Class
Green	Capsule	Abbott™ / Abbott™	Desbutal	methamphetamine / pentobarbital	5 / 30	
Green	Capsule		Placidyl	ethchlorvynol	750	Hypnotic
Green	Capsule	AHR 125	Tybatran	tybamate	125	Antianxiety
Green	Capsule	AHR 250	Tybatran	tybamate	250	
Green	Capsule	AHR 350	Tybatran	tybamate	350	Antianxiety
Green/two tone	Capsule	Pfizer 541	Vistaril	hydroxyzine	25	Antianxiety
Green/clear, dark green band (green yellow pellets)	Capsule	TUTAG	Cydril	levamphetamine	21	Stimulant
Green/clear, (green/white pellets)	Capsule	NAP	Amodril	levamphetamine	21	Stimulant
	Capsule	SKF D91 (1 dot)	Dexamyl	dextroamphetamine / amobarbital	10 / 65	
	Capsule	SKF D92 (2 dots)	Dexamyl	dextroamphetamine / amobarbital	15 / 97	
Green/black	Capsule	Stasenburgh™ 18-899	Biphetamine-T 12½	dextroamphetamine / amphetamine / methaqualone	6.25 / 6.25 / 40	
Green/black	Capsule	ROCHE 2	Librium	chlordiazepoxide	10	Antianxiety
Green/blue (turquoise)	Capsule	P-D 572	Parest	methaqualone	200	Hypnotic

Color	Shape/form	Special marks[a]	Trade name	Chemical composition	Dosage (mg)	Drug type[c]
Green/blue	Capsule	P-D 574	Parest	methaqualone	400	Hypnotic
Green/gray	Capsule	Pfizer 543	Vistaril	hydroxyzine	100	Antianxiety
Green/white	Capsule		Butatrax	amobarbital butabarbital	20 30	Sedative
		MCNEIL	Buticaps	butabarbital	30	Sedative
		McKesson[TM]	Kessodanten	diphenylhydantoin	100	Anticonvulsant
		ROCHE 3	Librium	chlordiazepoxide	25	Antianxiety
		Pfizer 542	Vistaril	hyroxyzine	50	Antianxiety
Green/yellow	Capsule	USV[TM]	Dexaspan-B	dextroamphetamine amobarbital	15 100	
		ROCHE 1	Librium	chlordiazepoxide	5	Antianxiety
Orange						
Orange	Ovoid Cap	Lederle[TM] 10 mg Lederle[TM] 15 mg	Dexa-Sequels Dexa-Sequels	dextroamphetamine dextroamphetamine	10 15	Stimulant Stimulant
Orange	Capsule	Lilly F72 30 mg	Seconal	secobarbital	30	Sedative
Orange	Capsule	Lilly F42 50 mg	Seconal	secobarbital	50	Sedative
Orange	Capsule	Lilly F40 100 mg	Seconal	secobarbital	100	Sedative
Orange	Capsule	P-D 237	Zarontin	ethosuximide	250	Anticonvulsant
Orange (orange band)	Capsule	P-D 393	Milontin	phensuximide	500	Anticonvulsant
Orange (two-tone)	Capsule	Lederle[TM]	Bamadex	dextroamphetamine	15	

Color	Form	Code	Trade name	Generic	mg	Category
Orange/blue	Capsule			meprobamate	300	⎫
Orange/blue		Lilly TM F64	Tuinal	secobarbital / amobarbital	25 / 25	⎬ Hypnotic
Orange/blue	Capsule	Lilly TM F65	Tuinal	secobarbital / amobarbital	50 / 50	Hypnotic
Orange/blue	Capsule	Lilly F66	Tuinal	secobarbital / amobarbital	100 / 100	⎭ Hypnotic
Orange/clear (orange/white pellets)	Capsule	SKF T63 (1 dot)	Thorazine	chlorpromazine	30	Antipsychotic
		SKF T64 (2 dots)	Thorazine	chlorpromazine	75	
		SKF T66 (3 dots)	Thorazine	chlorpromazine	150	
		SKF T67 (4 dots)	Thorazine	chlorpromazine	200	
		SKF T69 (5 dots)	Thorazine	chlorpromazine	300	
Orange/gray	Capsule	Obedrin	methamphetamine pentobarbital vitamins	5 / 20		
Orange/white	Capsule	McNeil	Buticaps	butabarbital	50	Sedative
Orange/white	Capsule	ROCHE 65	Dalmane	flurazepam	15	Hypnotic
Orange/white	Capsule	5 mg 573	Navane	thiothixene	5	Antipsychotic
Orange/white, red band	Capsule	P-D 399	Milontin	phensuximide	250	Anticonvulsant
Orange/yellow	Capsule	1 mg 571	Navane	thiothixene	1	Antipsychotic
		USV TM	Dexaspan	dextroamphetamine	15	Stimulant

Pink

Color	Form	Code	Trade name	Generic	mg	Category
Pink (flesh)	Capsule	Rowell	Lithonate	lithium carbonate	300	Antimanic
Pink	Capsule	Geigy TM 05	Pertofrane	desipramine	25	Antidepressant
Pink, (two tone)	Capsule	Pfizer 50 536	Sinequan	doxepin	50	Antidepressant
Pink/turquoise	Capsule	Pfizer 25 535	Sinequan	doxepin	25	Antidepressant

Color	Shape/form	Special marks[a]	Trade name	Chemical composition	Dosage (mg)	Drug type[c]
Pink/maroon	Capsule	Geigy^TM 07	Pertofrane	desipramine	50	Antidepressant
Pink/red	Capsule	Pfizer 10 534	Sinequan	doxepin	10	Antidepressant
Pink/white	Capsule	MCNEIL WYETH 10	Buticaps Serax	butabarbital oxazepam	100 10	Sedative Antianxiety
Purple	Capsule	W	Lotusate	talbutal	120	Sedative
Purple/clear (pink/white pellets)	Capsule	SKF A90	Benzedrine Spansule	amphetamine	15	Stimulant
Purple (lavender)/white	Capsule	McNEIL	Buticaps	butabarbital	15	Sedative
Purple (amythest)/white	Capsule	ROCHE 19	Noludar	methyprylon	300	Hypnotic
Purple (maroon)/white	Capsule	WYETH 30	Serax	oxazepam	30	Antianxiety
Purple (maroon)/pink	Capsule	Geigy 07	Pertofrane	desipramine	50	Antidepressant
Red						
Red	Round capsule		Paradione 150 Paradione 300	paramethadione paramethadione	150 300	Anticonvulsant Anticonvulsant
Red	Round capsule		Placidyl 100 Placidyl 200 Placidyl 500	ethchlorvynol ethchlorvynol ethchlorvynol	100 200 500	Hypnotic Hypnotic Hypnotic

Color	Type	Manufacturer	Brand	Drug	Strength	Category
Red	Capsule	McKESSON	Kessodrate 250	chloral hydrate	250	Sedative
		McKESSON	Kessodrate 500	chloral hydrate	500	Sedative
		Squibb 623	Noctec 250	chloral hydrate	250	Sedative
		Squibb 626	Noctec 500	chloral hydrate	500	Sedative
		FELLOWS 730	Paral	paraldehyde	975	Sedative
Red/black	Capsule	Strasenburgh™	Biphetamine T20	dextroamphetamine amphetamine methaqualone	10 10 40	
Red/clear (white pellets)	Capsule		PERKé ONE	dextroamphetamine	15	Stimulant
Red/clear (red/white pellets)	Capsule		Equanil LA	meprobamate	400	Antianxiety
Red/pink	Capsule	Pfizer 10 534	Sinequan	doxepin	10	Antidepressant
Red/white	Capsule	ROCHE 66	Dalmane	flurazepam	30	Hypnotic
		WYETH 15	Serax	oxazepam	15	Antianxiety
Red/yellow, clear	Capsule		PERKé TWO	dextroamphetamine amobarbital	15 60	
Red/yellow	Capsule	Fellows Testagar™ 045	Amodex Junior	dextroamphetamine amobarbital	7.5 30	
White						
White	Capsule	Strasenburgh™ 18-895	Biphetamine 7½	amphetamine dextroamphetamine	3.75 3.75	Stimulant
		Abbott™	Tridione	trimethadione	300	Anticonvulsant
White, black band	Capsule	P-D 531	Dilantin with Phenobarbital	diphenylhydantoin phenobarbital	100 32.5	Anticonvulsant

Color	Shape/form	Special marks[a]	Trade name	Chemical composition	Dosage (mg)	Drug type[c]
White, blue band	Capsule	P-D 372	Carbrital	pentobarbital carbromal	97.5 260	Sedative
		P-D 376	Carbrital	pentobarbital carbromal	48.5 130	
White, orange band	Capsule	P-D 362	Dilantin	diphenylhydantoin	100	Anticonvulsant
White, light orange band	Capsule	P-D 385	Dilantin D-A	diphenylhydantoin	100	Anticonvulsant
White, pink band	Capsule	P-D 365	Dilantin	diphenylhydantoin	30	Anticonvulsant
White, red band	Capsule	P-D 375	Dilantin with Phenobarbital	diphenylhydantoin phenobarbital	100 16	Anticonvulsant
White/black	Capsule	Strasenburgh[TM] 18-878	Biphetamine 12½	dextroamphetamine amphetamine	6.25 6.25	Stimulant
White/blue	Capsule	400	Felsules	chloral hydrate	244	Sedative
		Adipex Ty-Med		methamphetamine amobarbital	10 50	
White/blue	Capsule	CIBA	Doriden	glutethimide	500	Hypnotic
White/blue (aqua)	Capsule	10 mg 574	Navane	thiothixene	10	Antipsychotic
White/clear, black band (gray pellets)	Capsule	Reid-Provident[TM]	Toin Unicelles	diphenylhydantoin	250	Anticonvulsant
White/green	Capsule	ROCHE 3	Librium	chlordiazepoxide	25	Antianxiety
		Pfizer 542	Vistaril	hydroxyzine	50	

Color	Form	Marking	Trade name	Generic	Dose (mg)	Category
White/orange	Capsule		Butatrax	amobarbital	20	Sedative
				butabarbital	30	
		MCNEIL	Buticaps	butabarbital	30	Sedative
		McKesson^{TM}	Kessodanten	diphenylhydantoin	100	Anticonvulsant
White/orange, red band	Capsule	MCNEIL	Buticaps	butabarbital	50	Sedative
		ROCHE 65	Dalmane	flurazepam	15	Hypnotic
		5 mg 573	Navane	thiothixene	5	Antipsychotic
		P-D 399	Milontin	phensuximide	250	Anticonvulsant
White/pink	Capsule	MCNEIL	Buticaps	butabarbital	100	Sedative
White/purple (lavender)	Capsule	MCNEIL	Buticaps	butabarbital	15	Sedative
White/purple (amythest)	Capsule	ROCHE 19	Noludar	methyprylon	300	Hypnotic
White/purple (maroon)	Capsule	WYETH 30	Serax	oxazepam	30	Antianxiety
		WYETH 15	Serax	oxazepam	15	Antianxiety
White/red	Capsule	ROCHE 66	Dalmane	flurazepam	30	Hypnotic
White/yellow	Capsule	Lilly^{TM} H17	Aventyl	nortriptyline	10	Antidepressant
		Lilly^{TM} H19	Aventyl	nortriptyline	25	Antidepressant

Yellow

Color	Form	Marking	Trade name	Generic	Dose (mg)	Category
Yellow	Ovoid capsule		Solacen	Tybamate	250	Antianxiety
			Solacen	Tybamate	350	Antianxiety
Yellow	Capsule-shaped	FELLOWS 410	Felsules	chloral hydrate	65	Sedative
Yellow	Capsule	Abbott^{TM}	Nembutal	sodium pentobarbital	30	Sedative
		Abbott^{TM}	Nembutal	sodium pentobarbital	100	Sedative
Yellow, brown band	Capsule	P-D 537	Celontin	methsuximide	150	Anticonvulsant

Color	Shape/form	Special marks[a]	Trade name	Chemical composition	Dosage (mg)	Drug type[c]
Yellow, orange band	Capsule	P-D 525	Celontin	methsuximide	300	Anticonvulsant
Yellow, orange band	Capsule	P-D 394	Phelantin	phenobarbital	30	
				diphenylhydantoin	100	
				methamphetamine	2.5	
Yellow/aqua	Capsule	572 (2 mg)	Navane	thiothixene	2	Antipsychotic
Yellow/blue	Capsule		EKKo Jr.	diphenylhydantoin	100	Anticonvulsant
	Capsule		EKKo Sr.	diphenylhydantoin	250	Anticonvulsant
Yellow/brown	Capsule-shaped	Fellows Testagar™	Amodex	dextroamphetamine	15	
Yellow/clear	Capsule	050		amobarbital	60	
Yellow/clear (yellow/white pellets)	Capsule	WALLACE 200	Meprospan	meprobamate	200	Antianxiety
Yellow/clear	Capsule	Abbott™	Nembutal	sodium pentobarbital	50	Sedative
Yellow/green	Capsule	USV™	Dexaspan-B	dextroamphetamine	15	
				amobarbital	100	
Yellow/green	Capsule	ROCHE 1	Librium	chlordiazepoxide	5	Antianxiety
Yellow/grey	Capsule	SKF JO7	Eskalith	lithium carbonate	300	Antimanic
Yellow/orange	Capsule	USV™	Dexaspan	dextroamphetamine	15	Stimulant
Yellow/orange	Capsule	571 (1 mg)	Navane	thiothixene	1	Antipsychotic
Yellow/red	Capsule-shaped	Fellows Testagar™	Amodex Jr.	dextroamphetamine	7.5	
				amobarbital	30	
Yellow, clear/red	Capsule	045	PERKE Two	dextroamphetamine	15	
				amobarbital	60	
Yellow/white	Capsule	Lilly™ H17	Aventyl	nortriptyline	10	Antidepressant
		Lilly™ H19	Aventyl	nortriptyline	25	Antidepressant

RESTRICTED FOODS FOR
PATIENTS ON MAO INHIBITORS

	Tyramine content		
Food	High	Medium	Low
Cheeses			
Camembert	X		
Cheddar	X		
Gruyere	X		
Stilton	X		
Boursalt	X		
Emmenthal		X	
Brie		X	
Cracker Barrel-Kraft		X	
Blue		X	
Roquefort		X	
Romano		X	
American			X
Gouda			X
Parmesan			X

	Tyramine content		
Food	High	Medium	Low
Beverages			
Chianti wine	X		
Sherry wine		X	
Beer		X	
Riesling wine			X
Santeone wine			X
Champagne			X
Italian red wine (other than chianti)			X
Fish			
Pickled herring and lox	X		
Salted, dry herring		X	
Meat			
Chicken livers		X	

Other Restrictions

Fruits and vegetables
Canned figs
Raisins
Broad beans (fava beans)

Miscellaneous
Yeast products
Soy sauce
Yeast extracts
Chocolate
Excessive caffeine
Pickles/Sauerkraut

Other drugs also contraindicated, especially:
Amphetamines
Over-the-counter cold or hay fever preparations
Weight-reducing agents

DRUG ORDER CODES

Frequency or route	Code
Daily or once a day	OD
Every night	ON
At bedtime	HS
2 times a day	BID
3 times a day	TID
4 times a day	QID
Immediately (usually given only once)	STAT
Whenever necessary	PRN
Every half hour	Q1/2H
Every hour	QH
Every 2 hours	Q2H
Every 3 hours, etc.	Q3H, etc.
2 times a week	BIW
Every week	QW
Every 2 weeks	Q2W
Every 3 weeks, etc.	Q3W, etc.
Every 10 days	Q10Day
By mouth	PO
Intramuscular	IM
Intravenous	IV

REFERENCES

American Psychiatric Association. "Diagnostic and Statistical Manual: Mental Disorders." (2nd ed.) (DSM-II). Washington, D.C., 1968.

Annell, A. L. Lithium in the treatment of children and adolescents, *Acta Psychiatrica Scandinavica Suppl.*, 1969, **207**, 19–33.

Balance, W. D. G., Hirschfield, P. P., & Bringmann, W. G. Mental illness: Myth, metaphor, or model. *Professional Psychology*, 1970, **1**, 133–137.

Ban, T. A.: *Psychopharmacology.* Baltimore: Williams and Wilkins, 1969.

Bidder, T. G., Strain, J. J., & Brunschwig, L. Bilateral and unilateral ECT. Follow-up study and critique, *American Journal of Psychiatry*, 1970, **127**, 737–745.

Brill, N. Q., Koegler, R. R., Epstein, L. J., & Forgy, E. W. Controlled study of psychiatric outpatient treatment. *Archives of General Psychiatry*, 1964, **10**, 581–595.

Caffey, E. M., Diamond, L. S., Frank, T. V., Grasberger, J. C., Herman, L., Klett, C. J., & Rothstein, C. Discontinuation or reduction of chemotherapy in chronic schizophrenics. *Journal of Chronic Diseases*, 1964, **17**, 347–358.

Caffey, E. M., Hollister, L. E., Klett, C. J., & Kaim, S. C.: Veterans Administration (VA) Cooperative Studies in Psychiatry. In W. G. Clark and J. del Giudice (Eds.) *Principles of psychopharmacology.* New York: Academic Press, 1970.

Cannicott, S. M., & Waggoner, R. W. Comparative study of unilateral and bilateral ECT. *Archives of General Psychiatry*, 1967, **16**, 229–232.

Casey, J. F., Bennett, I. F., Lindley, C. J., Hollister, L. E., Gordon, M. H., & Springer, N. N. Drug therapy in schizophrenia. A controlled study of the effectiveness of chlorpromazine, promazine, phenobarbital, and placebo. *Archives of General Psychiatry*, 1960, **2**, 210–220. (a)

Casey, J. F., Lasky, J. J., Klett, C. J., & Hollister, L. E. Treatment of schizophrenic reactions with phenothiazine derivatives. A comparative study of chlorpromazine, triflupromazine, mepazine, prochlorperazine, perphenazine and pheno-barbital. *American Journal of Psychiatry*, 1960, **117**, 97–105. (b)

Casey, J. F., Hollister, L. E., Klett, C. J., Lasky, J. J., & Caffey, E. M. Combined drug therapy of chronic schizophrenics. Controlled evaluation of placebo, dextro-amphetamine, imipramine, isocarboxazid and trifluoperazine added to maintenance doses of chlorpromazine. *American Journal of Psychiatry*, 1961, **117**, 997–1003.

Chien, C-P. Psychiatric treatment for geriatric patients: "Pub" or drug? *American Journal of Psychiatry*, 1971, **127**, 1070–1075.

Clark, W. G. and del Giudice, J. (Eds.): *Principles of Psychopharmacology*. New York: Academic Press, 1970.

Cohen, B. D., Noblin, C. D., Silverman, A. J., & Penick, S. B. Functional asymmetry of the human brain. *Science*, 1968, **162**, 475–477.

Conners, C. K.: Review of stimulant drugs in learning and behavior disorders. *Psychopharmacology Bulletin*, 1971, **7**, 39–40.

Conners, C. K., Rothschild, G., Eisenberg, L., Schwartz, L. J., & Robinson, E., Dextroamphetamine sulfate in children with learning disorders. *Archives of General Psychiatry*, 1969, **21**, 182–190.

Crane, G. E. Tardive dyskinesia in patients treated with major neuroleptics. A review of the literature. *American Journal of Psychiatry Suppl.*, 1968, **124**, 40–48.

Dole, V., & Nyswander, M. Methadone maintenance. A report of two years' experience. In *Problems of drug dependence*. Washington, D.C.: National Academy of Science, National Research Council, 1966. Pp. 4611–4624.

Eveloff, H. H. Pediatric psychopharmacology. In W. G. Clark and J. del Giudice (Eds), *Principles of psychopharmacology*. New York: Academic Press, 1970.

Fink, M. *et al.* Naloxone in opiate dependence. In *Problems of drug abuse*. Washington, D.C.: Academy of Sciences, National Research Council, 1968. Pp. 5306–5313.

Fish, B. The importance of diagnostic syndromes in the drug treatment of hyper-kinesis. *Psychopharmacology Bulletin*, 1971, **7**, 39–40.

Fish, B. The "One Child, One Drug" myth of stimulants in hyperkinesis. Importance of diagnostic categories in evaluating treatment. *Archives of General Psychiatry*, 1971, **25**, 193–203.

Fleminger, J. J., Horne, DeL, Nair, N. P. V., & Nott, P. N. Differential effect of unilateral and bilateral ECT. *American Journal of Psychiatry*, 1970, **127**, 430–436.

Freedman, A. M. Drug addiction: An eclectic view. In *Problems of drug dependence*. Washington, D.C.: National Academy of Science, National Research Council, 1966, Pp. 4633–4640.

Frommer, E. A. Depressive illness in childhood. *British Journal of Psychiatry Spec. Publ.*, 1968, **2**, 117–136.

Gattozzi, A. A. *Lithium in the treatment of mood disorders*. Washington, D.C.: National Institute of Mental Health, 1970, Publ. No. 5033.

Gayral, L. and Lambert, P. La dichlorhydrate de fluphenazine. Etude des doses elèves et des traitments de longue dureé. *Proceedings of the 5th International Congress of Neuropsychopharmacology, Washington, D.C., 1966.* Amsterdam: Excerpta Medica Foundation, International Congress Series No. 129, 1967. Pp. 1128–1134.

General Practitioner Research Group. Phenobarbitone compared with an inactive placebo in anxiety states. *Practitioner,* 1964, **192,** 147–151.

Gershon, S. and Shopsin, B. (Eds.) *Lithium. Its role in psychiatric research and treatment.* New York: Plenum Press, 1972.

Gittelman-Klein, R. and Klein, D. F. Controlled imipramine treatment of school phobia. *Archives of General Psychiatry,* 1971, **25,** 204–207.

Goldberg, S. C. Brief resumé of the National Institute of Mental Health Study in Acute Schizophrenia. In W. G. Clark & J. del Giudice (Eds.) *Principles of Psychopharmacology.* New York: Academic Press, 1970.

Goldberg, S. C., Mattsson, N., Cole, J. O., & Klerman, G. L. Prediction of improvement in schizophrenia under four phenothiazines. *Archives of General Psychiatry,* 1967, **16,** 107–117.

Gorham, D. R., & Pokorny, A. D. Effects of phenothiazine and/or group psychotherapy with schizophrenics. *Diseases of the Nervous System,* 1964, **25,** 77–86.

Greenblatt, M., Grosser, G. H., & Wechsler, H. A comparative study of selected antidepressant medications and EST. *American Journal of Psychiatry,*1962, **119,** 144–153.

Greenblatt, M., Grosser, G. H., & Wechsler, H. Differential response of hospitalized depressed patients to somatic therapy. *American Journal of Psychiatry,* 1964, **120,** 935–943.

Greenblatt, M., Solomon, M. H., Evans, A. S., & Brooks, G. W. (Eds.) *Drug and social therapy in chronic schizophrenia.* Springfield, Ill.: Charles C. Thomas, 1965.

Grinspoon, L., Ewalt, J. R., & Shader, R.: Psychotherapy and pharmacotherapy in chronic schizophrenia. *American Journal of Psychiatry,* 1968, **124,** 1645–1652.

Heinicke, C. M. Parental deprivation in early childhood: A predisposition to later depression? Paper presented at Animal Behavior Society, Chicago, December 1970.

Hoffer, A., Osmond, H., Calbeck, M. J. *et al.* Treatment of schizophrenia with nicotinic acid and nicotinamide. *Journal of Clinical & Experimental Psychopathology,* 1957, **18,** 131–158.

Holliday, A. R. Review of psychopharmacology. In B. B. Wolman (Ed.) *Handbook of clinical psychology.* New York: McGraw-Hill, 1965, Pp. 1296–1322.

Hollister, L. E. Choice of antipsychotic drugs. *American Journal of Psychiatry,* 1970, **127**: 186–190.

Hollister, L. E. & Kosek, C. Sudden death during treatment with phenothiazine derivatives. *Journal of the American Medical Association,* 1965, **192,** 1035–1038.

Honigfeld, G. Non-specific factors in treatment. I. Review of placebo reactions and placebo reactors. *Diseases of the Nervous System,* 1964, **25,** 145–156. (a)

Honigfeld, G.: Non-specific factors in treatment. II. Review of social psychological factors. *Diseases of the Nervous System*, 1964, **25**, 225–239. (b)

Honigfeld, G. Specific and non-specific factors in the treatment of depressed state. In Rickels, K. (Ed.) *Non-specific factors in drug therapy*. Springfield, Ill. Charles C. Thomas, 1968. Pp. 80–107.

Honigfeld, G., Gillis, R. D., & Klett, C. J. NOSIE-30: A treatment sensitive ward behavior scale. *Psychological Reports*, 1966, **19**, 180–182.

Honigfeld, G., Klein, D. F., & Feldman, S. Prediction of psychopharmacologic effect in man: Development and validation of a computerized diagnostic decision tree. *Computers & Biomedical Research*, 1969, **2**, 350–361.

Honigfeld, G., & Klett, C. J. The nurse's observation scale for impatient evaluation. A new ward behavior rating scale. *Journal of Clinical Psychology*, 1965, **21**, 65–71.

Honigfeld, G., Rosenblum, M. P., Blumenthal, I. J., Lambert, H. L., & Roberts, A. J. Behavioral improvement in the older schizophrenic patient: Drug and social therapies. *Journal of the American Geriatrics Society*, 1965, **8**, 57–72.

Hornykiewicz, O., Markham, C. H., Clark, W. G., & Fleming, R. M. Mechanisms of extra-pyramidal side effects of therapeutic agents. In W. G. Clark & J. del Giudice (Eds.) *Principles of psychopharmacology*. New York: Academic Press, 1970.

Jaffe, J. Psychopharmacology and opiate dependence. In *Psychopharmacology: A review of progress*. Proceedings of the 6th Annual Meeting of the American College of Neuropsychopharmacology, December 1967. Public Health Service, 1968. Publication No. 1836.

Jenner, F. A., Kerry, R. J., & Parkin, D. A controlled comparison of methaminodiazepoxide (chlordiazepoxide, "Librium") and amylobarbitone in the treatment of anxiety in neurotic patients. *Journal of Mental Science*, 1961, **107**: 583–589.

Johnson, G., Gershon, S., & Hekimian, L. Controlled evaluation of lithium and chlorpromazine in the treatment of manic states. An interim report. *Comprehensive Psychiatry*, 1968, **9**, 563–573.

Kaim, S. C., Klett, C. J., & Rothfeld, B. Treatment of the acute alcohol withdrawal state. A comparison of four drugs. Perry Point, Maryland: Central Neuropsychiatric Research Lab., Report No. 72, August 1968.

Kalant, O. J.: *The amphetamines: Toxicity and addiction*. Springfield, Ill.: Charles C. Thomas, 1966.

Katz, M. M., Cole, J. O., & Barton, W. E. (Eds.) *The role and methodology of classification in psychiatry and psychopathology*. U.S. Govt. Printing Office, Washington, D. C.: Public Health Publ. No. 1584, 1968.

Klein, D. F. Importance of psychiatric diagnosis in prediction of clinical drug effects. *Archives of General Psychiatry*, 1967, **16**, 118–126.

Klein, D. F. Psychiatric diagnosis and a typology of clinical drug effects. *Psychopharmacologia*, 1968, **13**, 359–386.

Klein, D. F., & Davis, J. M. *Diagnosis and drug treatment of psychiatric disorders.* Baltimore: Williams and Wilkins, 1969

Klein, D. F., Honigfeld, G., & Feldman, S. Prediction of drug effect by a successive screening, decision tree diagnostic technique. In P. R. A. May & J. R. Wittenborn (Eds.) *Psychotropic drug response: Advances in prediction.* Springfield, Ill.: Charles C. Thomas, 1969. Pp. 45–91.

Klein, D. F., & Howard, A. *The psychiatric case study: Treatment, drugs and outcome.* Baltimore: Williams and Wilkins, 1972.

Klerman, G. L. Clinical efficacy and actions of antipsychotics. In A. DiMascio & R. I. Shader (Eds.) *Clinical handbook of psychopharmacology* New York: Science House, 1970.

Klerman, G. L., & Paykel, E. S. The tricyclic antidepressants. In W. G. Clark & J. del Giudice (Eds.) *Principles of psychopharmacology.* New York: Academic Press, 1970.

Klett, C. J., & Moseley, E. C. The right drug for the right patient. *Journal of Consulting Psychology,* 1965, **29**, 546–551.

Leetsma, J. E., & Koenig, K. L. Sudden death and phenothiazines: A current controversy. *Archives of General Psychiatry,* 1968, **18**, 137–148.

Lifshitz, K., & Kline, N. S. Psychopharmacology in geriatrics. In W. G. Clark & J. del Giudice (Eds.) *Principles of psychopharmacology.* New York: Academic Press, 1970. Pp. 695–705.

Lusted, L. B., & Stahl, W. R. Conceptual models of diagnosis. In R. Kleinmuntz (Ed.) *Clinical information processing by computer.* New York: Holt, 1969.

Maggs, R. Treatment of manic illness with lithium carbonate. *British Journal of Psychiatry,* 1963, **109**, 56–65..

Mark. V. H., & Ervin, F. R. *Violence and the brain.* New York: Harper & Row, 1970.

Marks, I. M. *Fears and phobias.* New York: Academic Press, 1969.

Martin, W. R. The basis and possible utility of the use of opioid antagonists in the ambulatory treatment of the addict. In A. Wikler (Ed.) *The addictive states,* Baltimore: Williams and Wilkins, 1968. Pp. 367–371.

May, P. R. A. *Treatment of schizophrenia.* New York: Science House, 1968.

Monroe, R. R. *Episodic behavioral disorders.* Boston: Harvard Univ. Press, 1970.

Nathan, P. E. *Cues, decisions and diagnoses.* New York: Academic Press, 1967.

Osmond, H., & Hoffer, A. Massive niacin treatment in schizophrenia. Review of a nine year study. *Lancet,* 1962, **1**, 316–320.

Overall, J. E. & Gorham, D. R. The brief psychiatric rating scale. *Psychological Reports,* 1962, **10**, 799–812.

Overall, J. E., Hollister, L. E., Pokorny, A. D., Casey, J. F., & Katz, G. Drug therapy in depressions. Controlled evaluation of imipramine, isocarboxazid dextroamphetamine-amobarbital and placebo. *Clinical Pharmacology and Therapeutics* 1962, **3**, 16–22.

Polvan, N., Yagcioglu, V., Itil, T., *et al.* High and very high dose fluphenazine in the treatment of chronic psychosis. Amsterdam: Excerpta Medica Foundation, International Congress Series, No. 180, 1969. Pp. 495–497.

Prange, A. J., Wilson, I. C., Knox, A., McClane, T. K., & Lipton, M. Enhancement of imipramine by thyroid stimulating hormone: Clinical and theoretical implications. *American Journal of Psychiatry*, 1970, **127**, 191–199.

Prien, R. F., Caffey, E. M., & Klett, C. J. Lithium carbonate: A survey of the history and current status of lithium in treating mood disorders. *Diseases of the Nervous System*, 1971, **32**, 521–531.

Prien, R. F., Caffey, E. M., & Klett, C. J. Lithium carbonate in psychiatry. Washington, D. C.: American Psychiatric Association, 1970.

Prien, R. F., Caffey, E. M., & Klett, C. J. A comparison of lithium carbonate and chlorpromazine in the treatment of mania. *Archives of General Psychiatry*, 1972, **26**, 146–153. (a)

Prien, R. F., Caffey, E. M., & Klett, C. J. A comparison of lithium carbonate and chlorpromazine in the treatment of excited schizo-affectives. *Archives of General Psychiatry*, 1972, **27**, 182–193. (b).

Prien, R. R., & Cole, J. O. High dose chlorpromazine therapy in chronic schizophrenia. *Archives of General Psychiatry*, 1968, **18**, 482–495.

Prien, R. F., & Klett, C. J. An appraisal of the long term use of tranquilizing medication with hospitalized chronic schizophrenics. A review of the drug discontinuation literature. *National Institute of Mental Health Schizophrenia Bulletin*, 1972.

Prien, R. F., Levine, J., & Cole, J. O. High dose trifluoperazine therapy in chronic schizophrenia. *American Journal of Psychiatry*, 1969, **126**, 305–313.

Prien, R. F., Levine, J., & Switalski, R. W. Discontinuation of chemotherapy in chronic schizophrenia: Results from two collaborative studies. *Hospital and Community Psychiatry*, 1971, **22**, 20–23.

Quitkin, F. & Rifkin, A: Phobic anxiety syndrome complicated by drug dependence and addiction: A treatable form of drug abuse. *Archives of General Psychiatry*, 1972, **27**, 159–162.

Quitkin, F. M., Rifkin, A., & Klein, D. F. Lithium and other psychiatric disorders. In S. Gershon & B. Shopsin (Eds.) *Lithium: Its role in psychiatric research and treatment*. New York: Plenum Press, 1972.

Rech, R. H., & Moore, K. F. (Eds.) *An introduction to psychopharmacology*. New York: Raven Press, 1971.

Reynolds, E., Joyce, C. R. B., Swift, J. L., Tooley, P. H., & Weatherall, M. Psychological and clinical investigation of the treatment of anxious outpatients with three barbiturates and placebo. *British Journal of Psychiatry*, 1965, **111**, 84–95.

Rifkin, A., Levitan, S., Galewski, J., & Klein, D. F. Emotionally unstable character disorders: A follow-up study. I. Description of patients and outcome. II. Prediction of outcome. *Journal of Biological Psychiatry*, 1972, **4**, 65–88.(a)

Rifkin, A., Quitkin, F. M., Carillo, C., & Klein, D. F. Very high dosage fluphenazine for non-chronic, treatment-refractory patients. *Archives of General Psychiatry*, 1971, **25**, 398–403.

Rifkin, A., Quitkin, F., Carrillo, C., & Klein, D. F. Lithium treatment of emotionally unstable character disorders. Unpublished manuscript, 1972. (b)

Robin, A. A., & Harris, J. A. Controlled comparison of imipramine and electroplexy. *Journal of Mental Science*, 1962, **108**, 217–219.

Schlagenhauf, G., Tupin, J. P., & White, R. The use of lithium carbonate in the treatment of manic psychosis. *American Journal of Psychiatry*, 1966, **123**, 201–206.

Schou, M. Special review: Lithium in psychiatric therapy and prophylaxis. *Journal of Psychiatric Research*, 1968, **6**, 67–95.

Schou, M., Baastrup, P. C., Grof, P., Weis, P., & Angst., J. Pharmacological and clinical problems of lithium prophylaxis. *British Journal of Psychiatry*, 1970, **116**, 615–619.

Sharma, S. L. A historical background of the development of nosology in psychiatry and psychology. *American Psychologist*, 1970, **25**, 248–253.

Sletten, I. W., & Gershon, S. The premenstrual syndrome: A discussion of its pathophysiology and treatment with lithium. *Comprehensive Psychiatry*, 1966, **1**, 197–206.

Smith, M. E., & Chassan, J. B. Comparisons of diazepam, chlorpromazine and trifluoperazine in a double-blind clinical investigation. *Journal of Neuropsychiatry*, 1964, **5**, 593–600.

Spitzer, R. L., & Endicott, J. DIAGNO: A computer program for psychiatric diagnosis utilizing the differential diagnostic procedure. *Archives of General Psychiatry*, 1968, **18**, 746–756.

Strain, J. J., Brunschwig, L., Duffy, J. P., Angle, D. P., Rosenbaum, A. L., & Bidder, T. G. Comparison of therapeutic effects and memory changes with bilateral and unilateral ECT. *American Journal of Psychiatry*, 1968, **125**, 294–304.

Vilkin, M. I. Comparative chemotherapeutic trial in treatment of chronic borderline patients. *American Journal of Psychiatry*, 1964, **120**, 1004.

Wheatley, D. Chlordiazepoxide in the treatment of the domicilliary case of anxiety neurosis. *Proceedings of the 4th World Congress of Psychiatry*. Amsterdam: Excerpta Medica, 1968.

Wing, L., & Lader, M. H. Physiological and clinical effects of amylobarbitone sodium therapy in patients with anxiety states. *Journal of Neurology, Neurosurgery and Psychiatry*, 1965, **28**, 78–87.

SUBJECT INDEX

This index cites principally general categories of drugs; e.g., antipsychotic agents, MAO inhibitors, and antianxiety agents. However, some of the more popular drugs, and those of special interest are indexed by generic name. Comprehensive drug lists may be found in the appropriate appendixes or tables.

215

D 5
E 6
F 7
G 8
H 9
I 0
J 1
  2
  3